Master the Boards
USMLE® Medical Ethics

Third Edition

ALSO FROM KAPLAN MEDICAL

Books

USMLE™ Step 1 Qbook

Master the Boards USMLE™ Step 2 CK

USMLE™ Step 2 CK Qbook

USMLE™ Step 2 Clinical Skills

USMLE™ Step 2 CS: Complex Cases

Master the Boards USMLE™ Step 3

USMLE™ Step 3 Qbook

Master the Boards Internal Medicine

Internal Medicine Question Book

Flashcards

USMLE® Diagnostic Test Flashcards:
The 200 Questions You Need to Know for the Exam for Steps 2 & 3

USMLE® Examination Flashcards:
The 200 "Most Likely Diagnosis" Questions You Will See on the Exam for Steps 2 & 3

USMLE® Pharmacology and Treatment Flashcards:
The 200 Questions You're Most Likely to See on Steps 1, 2 & 3

USMLE® Physical Findings Flashcards:
The 200 Questions You're Most Likely to See on the Exam

Online

Dr. Conrad Fischer's Comprehensive Cases

Updated USMLE® Step 3 Qbank

Master the Boards
USMLE® Medical Ethics

THE ONLY USMLE ETHICS HIGH-YIELD REVIEW

Third Edition

Conrad Fischer, MD
Caterina Oneto, MD

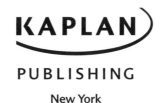

PUBLISHING

New York

© 2012 by Conrad Fischer, MD

Published by Kaplan Publishing, a division of Kaplan, Inc.
395 Hudson Street, 4th Floor
New York, NY 10014

Printed in the United States of America.

10 9 8 7 6 5 4 3 2 1

13-ISBN: 978-1-60714-904-0

Kaplan Publishing books are available at special quantity discounts to use for sales promotions, employee premiums, or educational purposes. For more information or to order books, please call the Simon & Schuster special sales department at 866-506-1949.

To:

Antonio Oneto
Lawyer, Politician, Humanist, Father, and Loyal Friend
A man of honor and integrity
C.O.

To:

Truth
C.F.

Contents

Introduction and How to Use This Book

Questions about medical ethics appear in the Behavioral Science section of Step 1 and in patient management in Step 3. Medical ethics topics account for half the Behavioral Science questions on Step 1 and are perceived as the most difficult questions on Step 3. This book will guide you through these challenging questions.

The book you have in your hands is a profoundly practical document that includes the most likely questions you will encounter on USMLE™, practice questions, and the most relevant text in the area of medical ethics.

This is not a book of philosophy. This book is to help you get the questions right on USMLE—all the questions.

Professional medical ethicists will not like our approach, which is to be concrete and definite. We avoid the "we'll see," "it depends," and other fuzzy, nonspecific pronouncements you might get on rounds. Professional ethicists do not have to answer "single best answer" standardized questions; you do.

We have made the questions specifically conservative enough that there is a definite correct answer—one that even ethicists will agree on.

If a subject is unlikely to appear on USMLE then you are unlikely to see it in this book. If we miss a subject, I would kindly appreciate you emailing me the subject within the confines of the confidentiality agreement of USMLE. We will add the subject and will be your friend for pointing out the deficiency.

This book includes a free 18-item medical ethics quiz, provided as an online companion. For access, log on to *kaptest.com/booksonline*. You will be asked for a password derived from the text to access the online companion, so have your book available.

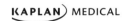

Please contact me at Conrad.Fischer@Touro.edu with any comments, questions, or disagreements. We have spent a long time making sure you have everything you need to answer the questions correctly for the test. As a by-product, you will also be on the very cutting edge of medical ethics and will be able to argue a point on rounds with any professional ethicists—and win.

Conrad Fischer, MD
Director of Educational Development, Department of Medicine
Jamaica Hospital
Associate Professor of Physiology, Pharmacology, and Medicine
Touro College of Osteopathic Medicine

Caterina Oneto, MD

About the Author

Conrad Fischer, MD, is director of educational development for the Department of Medicine at Jamaica Hospital Medical Center in New York City. Jamaica Hospital is a robust window on the world of medicine. Dr. Fischer is also chairman of medicine for Kaplan Medical, teaching USMLE Steps 1, 2, and 3, Internal Medicine Board Review and Attending Recertification, and USMLE Step 1 Physiology. Dr. Fischer is associate professor of physiology, pharmacology, and medicine at Touro College of Osteopathic Medicine in New York City.

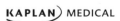

Chapter 1: **Autonomy**

Patient autonomy is the most fundamental principle underlying all health-care ethics. Autonomy grants every competent adult patient the absolute right to do what he wishes with his own health care. The concept of autonomy is fundamental to the entirety of the U.S. legal system and has complete acceptance as an operating principle of day-to-day decision making. Justice Cardozo set this as a clear legal precedent in 1914, in the case *Schloendorff v. Society of New York Hospital*, 105 N.E. 92 (1914). Justice Cardozo wrote, "Every human being of adult years and a sound mind has the right to determine what shall be done with his own body and a surgeon who performs an operation without his patient's consent commits an assault, for which he is liable in damages, except in cases of emergency where the patient is unconscious and where it is necessary to operate before consent can be obtained." Justice Cardozo was writing concerning the need for informed consent when a person undergoes surgery. In this case it was made clear that to perform surgery on a patient without his direct consent was equivalent to assault and battery.

Patient autonomy is a concept derived from the property rights issues that led to the Declaration of Independence, the U.S. Constitution, and the Bill of Rights. Autonomy over one's own medical care is seen in the same light as freedom of religion, freedom from illegal search and seizure, freedom of speech, and freedom of assembly. These rights are so intrinsic to our culture that they are considered axiomatic. Within the last 30 years they have been legally extended to cover the freedom to choose one's own form of health care. For example, patients have the right to refuse undesired therapy, and they have the right to choose whether or not they will participate in experimentation. Each patient has the right to have his wishes carried out even in the event that he loses consciousness or the capacity to make decisions for himself.

In part because treatments such as mechanical ventilation and artificial nutrition didn't exist in the past, we need new laws to delineate precisely the ethics of health care. Our ability to develop new forms of therapy has outpaced our ability to create ethical systems that determine whether or not these systems will be used in a specific case.

- Does the development and existence of a treatment—such as placement on a ventilator—mean we should always use it?
- Does the fact that we can place a nasogastric tube in a comatose patient and administer artificial nutrition that can keep that patient alive almost indefinitely mean we should do so?

Each patient should decide the answers to these questions for himself. This is autonomy: I have the right to do what I choose with my own body as long as I understand the consequences of my decisions. There is no form of property more personal than one's own body; so each patient has the right to determine what is done to his body. These principles may seem obvious, but they are fundamental in medical ethics. This work is an examination of the various ethical situations faced daily by physicians.

Autonomy represents a patient's right to determine his or her own health-care decisions. No form of a treatment can be pursued without his or her agreement, even if the proposed therapy is "for her own good." Although beneficence—or doing what is good for people—is a high aim and ethical principle, autonomy is considered more important and takes precedence. Each patient has the right to refuse a treatment even if that treatment has no adverse effects and will help her. You cannot treat him or her against his or her will even if the treatment is for her benefit.

Think of your body as a piece of property such as your house or your car. The police do not have the right to search your house at their whim. They must obtain a warrant. They cannot even do something benign, such as step inside your home, without your express agreement. Likewise, a physician cannot do a colonoscopy or a CBC without your consent. Unless you agree to it, a physician cannot even do a urinalysis or an EKG, even though these are mild and uncomplicated procedures.

Along the same lines, a painter cannot repaint your house without your consent even if he does it for free, the existing house color is ugly, and the service will only benefit you. A physician cannot treat your pneumonia or remove a cancer even though the procedure or treatment is benign and it will only benefit you.

A doctor can violate this autonomy if you are doing something potentially dangerous, such as building a bomb, because this activity can harm others. A doctor can violate your confidentiality only if you have HIV, tuberculosis, or a sexually transmitted disease because these conditions can harm an innocent third party. Your right to autonomy is only limited where there is potential harm to an innocent third party. Even in these cases, the violation of confidentiality is limited and tightly controlled.

The concept of patient autonomy is similar to that of voting. Ballot counters cannot make presumptions based on whom they think you will vote for. They must definitely know whom you intended to vote for when you were casting your vote. This must be based on whom you specifically voted for. Another person cannot bring your proxy ballot to the election based on which candidate he thinks you should vote for or which candidate will help you the most.

You must cast your vote in a manner based on your clearly stated wishes. You have a right to vote for the weakest candidate. You have the right to make the "wrong" choice. In the same way, a doctor can only render care for you based on what you tell her you want.

Patient autonomy gives you the right to make the wrong choice about your health care. Even if you are unable to make or express your health-care choices, the physician cannot simply make decisions for you that go against your wishes. This stands even if your choices would be harmful to you. This is one of the most difficult things for a physician to understand and act on. Doctors are trained to act in the best interest of their patients, but the patient's right to act against his own best interest comes first. Patients have the autonomy of free will.

Chapter 2: Competence and the Capacity to Make Decisions

DEFINITIONS

Competence is a legal term. Competency decisions transpire within the judicial system. Only a court can determine that a patient is incompetent. All adult patients are considered competent unless specifically proven otherwise. Physicians can determine whether or not a patient has the capacity to understand his medical condition.

The physician makes a determination of the capacity of a patient to comprehend her medical problems based on whether there is an organic delirium due to a medical condition such as a sodium problem, hypoxia, drug intoxication, meningitis, encephalitis, or a psychiatric disorder. These determinations are based in large part on a neurological examination testing memory, comprehension, reasoning, and judgment. Any physician can make this determination. The physician does not have to be a psychiatrist. A psychiatrist may be useful in rendering decision-making capacity determinations in cases that are complex or equivocal. If the patient obviously does or does not have the capacity to understand, a psychiatrist is not needed.

MINORS

By definition, a minor is a person under the age of 18. With some exceptions, minors are generally not considered competent to make their own decisions. Only a parent or a legal guardian can give consent for a minor. Neighbors, aunts, uncles, and grandparents cannot give consent for treatment of a minor. This rule does not cover life-threatening or serious emergencies. Consent is always implied for emergency treatment. A physician should not withhold blood or surgery in a life-threatening accident just because the parent is not present.

For example, a 10-year-old boy accidentally runs through a glass window at school and lacerates the radial artery. His teacher brings him to the emergency department. The boy is bleeding and needs both a blood transfusion and surgery to correct the defect. What should you do?

Emergency treatment of a minor does not need express written consent. Parental consent is implied. Saying that you had to ask another person such as the teacher, the principal, the school nurse, the babysitter, or the grandparents for consent before giving emergency treatment would be the wrong answer. Seeking a court order is also a wrong choice in an emergency because it delays the treatment and because in an emergency it is implied that the parents would consent if they were there.

Partial Emancipation

Although only a parent or guardian can give consent for procedures and therapies for a minor there are some exceptions to this rule in the areas of prenatal care, contraception, sexually transmitted diseases (STDs), and substance abuse. The mature minor is generally one above the age of 15, although this varies by state. USMLE will not make hairsplitting distinctions like giving you a 14-year-old the day before her 15th birthday. The case on the exam will be clear.

For example, a 16-year-old girl comes to see you in clinic to discuss contraception. She is generally healthy but is not accompanied by a parent. What should you do?

In all cases like this involving prenatal care, STDs, contraception, HIV and substance abuse the answer should be to treat the patient. Saying that you must notify the parents, get a court order, seek legal counsel, refuse therapy, or to go to the ethics committee are all incorrect answers. These interventions are not necessary. Society has an interest in preventing unwanted pregnancy, so it is considered less harmful to treat without parental notification than it is to take the risk that a teenager will get pregnant and need an abortion later.

Abortion in a Minor

The rules on parental notification for abortion are less clear because there is no national standard. Some states require parental notification and some don't.

For example, a 16-year-old girl comes to see you in her first trimester of pregnancy. She is seeking an abortion. What should you do?

In this case, there is no clear answer about whether or not the physician should notify the parents. There is no clear national standard and it depends upon the state you are in. The most likely right answer will indicate the need to encourage the child to notify the parents herself, which would be best. So the correct answer choice will say something like "encourage discussion," "counsel her to tell the parents herself," or "suggest a family meeting." On the ethics questions for USMLE, if there is a choice that says to discuss, confer, meet, or have voluntary notification, this will generally be the right thing to do first.

Emancipated Minor

A small number of minors, particularly at older ages such as 16 or 17, may be considered "emancipated" or freed of the need to have parental consent for any medical care. The criteria are that the minor is married, self-supporting and living independently, in the military, or the parent of a child that they themselves support. The criteria for being an emancipated minor relate to being no longer dependent on one's parents for support. In other words, if the minor does not live with his parents, has a job, and is self-supporting financially, then the minor no longer is dependent upon parental consent for his actions.

An emancipated minor is free to make health-care decisions in all areas, not only just STDs, prenatal care, contraception, or substance abuse. Serious medical conditions or procedures such as organ donation, surgery, or abortion may require a specific court order to allow the legal standing of emancipation to be fully valid. Only answer "court order," "judicial intervention," "court trial," or "seek legal resolution" if the case represents disagreement or a lack of consensus in the stem.

Limitations on Parental Right of Refusal for Minors

Although a competent adult can refuse any medical care she wishes, the same right does not automatically extend for parents concerning their children. Parents cannot refuse life-saving treatment for their child based on religious belief. The state has an interest in the welfare of the child that exceeds the parental right to deny therapy for the child if the child might die.

For example, a child is in a motor vehicle accident and sustains head trauma requiring surgery to drain a hematoma that, if left untreated, will be fatal. As part of the surgery the child will need a blood transfusion. The parents are Jehovah's Witnesses and refuse to give consent for the transfusion. The parents' stated religious beliefs are that accepting blood for their child would be a fate worse than death. What should you do?

If the child needs blood to save his life you must give the blood—even over the objection of the parents. It may seem contradictory to seek parental consent for a procedure that you will perform even if they refuse, but in this case, you should attempt to obtain their permission nonetheless.

Withholding lifesaving therapy for a child is considered comparable to child abuse. The parents' right to practice their religion in terms of health care would cover their ability to refuse a transfusion for themselves, but not for their child.

This ethical concept has only expanded. Parents cannot refuse therapy for children even if they are severely brain damaged or otherwise developmentally disabled. Society does not distinguish between individuals based on their relative 'worth.' In other words, parents cannot refuse tracheo-esophageal fistula repair on a patient with Down syndrome just because the mental capacity and functional ability of the child will be much less than that of a child without this disease. From this point of view, treatment against parents' wishes in a life-threatening situation is equally valid for both a future genius and a child with cerebral palsy who will not achieve a mental age above 2.

One of the only times parents are allowed to refuse care for their child is when the child is so ill or deformed that death is inevitable. This is not a true refusal on the part of the parent. This is really just saying that parents can refuse only the futile care that the doctor shouldn't be giving anyway.

PSYCHIATRIC PATIENTS

A patient's psychiatric history is intrinsic to the concept of competence and to the patient's capacity to understand her medical problems. A patient with the clear capacity to understand or one who clearly does not have capacity does not need a psychiatric evaluation. However, a psychiatric evaluation can be useful to help make a determination of capacity in equivocal or questionable cases.

All suicidal patients are considered to lack capacity to understand because active suicidal ideation is deemed to be a sign of impaired judgment. In addition, the level of competence necessary to make financial decisions is different from that necessary for an informed refusal. In other words, a patient may have a history of bipolar disorder making it impossible for him to manage his financial decisions. However, the same person might still be considered to have capacity to refuse treatment. There is a very limited demand placed on patients to establish capacity to refuse treatments.

CAPACITY TO REFUSE PROCEDURES IN AN OTHERWISE MENTALLY DISABLED PATIENT

A patient with mental illness or mental retardation that might be considered incompetent for other areas of life may still retain the right to refuse medical procedures. The criteria to determine competence in areas of finance are at a higher standard than those for refusing medical procedures. Your patient might have schizophrenia, mental retardation, or autism to the point of needing to live in a group home, but that does not mean they are incapable of understanding medical procedures. This means that an adult with a mental age of 8 or 10 may still be allowed to refuse medical procedures. Our society is reluctant to strap a patient to his bed and perform procedures that would be painful or uncomfortable for the patient without his consent. For instance, certain court cases in the past have allowed a patient with mental illness to refuse diagnostic procedures even though two out of three of the reasons for the refusal were delusional. This is an affirmation of how deep the principle of autonomy goes in the management of patients. In addition, it shows that beneficence—trying to do the right thing for patients—is considered less important than autonomy. Autonomy is given more weight in decision making than beneficence. Autonomy has priority.

A person may meet the legal standard of competence to refuse or accept medical care even if she is not considered competent in other areas of life, such as financial matters.

Chapter 3: **Informed Consent**

ALL OPTIONS MUST BE DESCRIBED

You must fully inform the patient of the risks and benefits of each procedure prior to undergoing the procedure. The explanation must be in language that the patient understands and include full information regarding alternative treatments. The patient cannot make an informed choice for one treatment if she does not know of the existence of others.

For example, you inform a patient about the risks and benefits of bone marrow transplantation for chronic myelogenous leukemia. You fully inform the patient about the risk of transplantation, including the possibility of developing graft versus host disease. After the transplantation the patient develops graft versus host disease, which is hard to control. The patient learns that there is an alternative treatment called imitanib (gleevec) which you did not tell them about. Gleevec does not include the risk of graft versus host disease, but will not cure the leukemia. The patient files suit against you. What will be the most likely outcome of the suit?

In this case the patient will probably win the suit because he was not fully informed about the alternatives to the therapies mentioned. The physician has an ethical duty to inform the patient about all the treatment options and then allow the patient to decide among them. Although the physician's preference of procedure or treatment may differ from what the patient chooses, the patient has the option to choose therapy that may not be what the doctor deems is best for him.

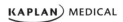

ALL MAJOR ADVERSE EFFECTS MUST BE DESCRIBED

Adverse effects and injury from medical care do not necessarily represent a mistake or failure of therapy. In the case described in the previous example, the error was not that graft versus host disease developed. The patient was fully informed that this could occur and he chose the bone marrow transplantation anyway. The error was not informing the patient of an alternative option in treatment. At the same time, a patient could potentially die as an adverse effect of treatment. This is only an ethical and legal problem if the adverse event happens and the patient was not told that it could have happened. The patient might say, "Doctor, I would never have taken digoxin if you had told me it might cause a rhythm disturbance or visual problem" or "I would never have had surgery if you had told me I might need a blood transfusion." The main point is to respect autonomy. The patient must be informed of the therapeutic options, the adverse effects of the procedure, and the harm of not undergoing the procedure. If they have the capacity to understand and they choose to do it anyway, they have made an autonomous therapeutic choice, and therefore, the patient bears the burden of any adverse effect, not the physician.

> *For example,* a man undergoes coronary angioplasty. He is informed that the artery may rupture and that there is a small chance he could bleed to death during the surgery to repair the damaged vessel. He knows he could have bypass surgery instead. He understands and chooses the angioplasty. He dies from a ruptured blood vessel. The family files suit against you. What will be the most likely outcome?

Although it is unfortunate that the patient died in this case, there is no liability with regard to informed consent or ethical error. The patient was informed of his treatment options and the possible complications, and he chose the treatment.

The patient must understand the risks of a procedure just as a driver must understand the risks before getting behind the wheel of a car. Why can't you sue a car manufacturer if you die in a car accident? Predominantly because you are an adult with the capacity to understand the risks of driving and you chose to drive anyway. The licensing process is an education process that both tries to make you a safe driver, while also properly informing you of the risks of driving. Each time you get in a car, there is implied consent that you are choosing the risk of driving. Even if you get into a car accident and are injured or killed, the manufacturer has no liability, as long as the car is well made, because as a competent adult you chose to put yourself at risk.

In addition to understanding the risks of the procedure, you must inform the patient of what could happen if she does not choose therapy that you offer.

> *For example,* a patient comes to the emergency department with appendicitis. He is informed of the risks of surgery, and refuses the procedure both verbally and in writing. The patient dies. What was done wrong here?

The patients must be informed both of the risk of the treatment as well as what will happen if they don't undergo the procedure. In this case the physician is liable in court because he never documented that he informed the patient of the possibility of appendiceal rupture and death if the patient did NOT have the procedure.

CONSENT IS REQUIRED FOR EACH SPECIFIC PROCEDURE

If the patient signs a consent form for an operation on her left knee, you cannot, in the operating room, decide to operate on her right knee and assume that you have consent. If a patient signs a consent for an appendectomy, but when you open her up you find colon cancer, you cannot just do the colectomy without first informing the patient of the additional procedure and obtaining her consent. There can be no presumption for consent for anything beyond what the patient specifically said she consented to. Either the patient has to sign consent in advance for the other procedures or she has to regain consciousness and have the additional procedure explained to her.

BENEFICENCE IS NOT SUFFICIENT TO ELIMINATE THE NEED FOR CONSENT

Trying to be sincere and to do good is very important and takes primacy; however, the patient's right to control what happens with his own body is more important.

> *For example,* a 40-year-old man is undergoing a nasal polypectomy. In the operating room you see a lesion on the nasal turbinate that the frozen section determines to be a cancer. You have found the cancer early but will need to resect the nasal turbinate to cure it. What should you do?

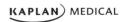

You cannot remove the cancerous lesion without the patient's approval. This is true even if the physician is sincere, talented, accurate, and helpful. This is true even if the procedure will save the patient's life, unless the illness is an emergency in an unconscious patient. Beneficence does not eliminate the need for informed consent. If you live in a very messy apartment your neighbor cannot break into your apartment to clean it even if he doesn't steal anything. You must consent to the cleaning. His good intentions are not as important as your right to do what you want with your own property.

DECISIONS MADE WHEN COMPETENT ARE VALID WHEN CAPACITY IS LOST

We must respect the last known wishes of a patient if she loses the capacity to communicate and state those wishes. Although it is preferable to have the patient's last known wishes documented in writing, following verbally expressed wishes is perfectly valid. Oral consent is valid for any level of procedure if the oral consent can be proven. The basis for validity of oral or written consent is not whether the procedure is large or small. In other words, it is not the case that oral consent is valid for a sigmoidoscopy but a brain biopsy requires written consent. A patient can give oral consent for a heart transplant if the patient is unable to write. The only difficulty is that if challenged, orally expressed wishes for treatment are more difficult to prove than written ones.

> *For example,* a 42-year-old man with leukemia repeatedly refuses chemotherapy. He loses consciousness and his mother tells you to give the chemotherapy. What should you tell her?

You must respect the last known wishes of the patient. If the patient does not want a treatment, you cannot just wait for him to lose consciousness and then perform the treatment. If this were permissible, then no one could have an estate will. The ultimate form of loss of decision-making capacity is death. We make out a will so that when we lose the capacity to speak for ourselves, our wishes for what to do with our property are respected after death.

> *For example,* a 64-year-old woman accompanied by her husband comes to the emergency room seeking treatment for chest pain. The patient clearly tells you that she wants to have her aorta repaired and she signs consent for the procedure. She later becomes hypotensive and loses consciousness. Her husband is now the decision maker and says, "Let her die." What do you tell him?

A patient's family member cannot wait for her to lose consciousness and then go against the patient's previously expressed wishes regarding treatments and procedures. In the case above, because the patient expressed that she would like to have her aorta repaired her husband cannot go against this after she loses consciousness. The same reasoning holds true if a patient refuses a procedure or treatment and then loses consciousness.

CONSENT IS IMPLIED IN AN EMERGENCY

For example, a 50-year-old construction worker arrives at the emergency room by ambulance after an accident lacerating his arm. He has lost so much blood he is unconscious. There is no family member available to sign consent. What should you do?

The management of an emergency is different. Consent is implied in an emergency for a patient without the capacity to speak for himself. This would not apply to a terminally ill patient with a pre-existing DNR order. Neither a court order, nor a hospital administrator, nor the ethics committee is required to give permission before the doctor can administer therapy in an emergency.

THE PERSON PERFORMING THE PROCEDURE SHOULD OBTAIN CONSENT

The person who is most knowledgeable about the procedure should obtain informed consent. Because we must inform the patient about all the options of treatment, risks of the options, and risks of not performing the procedure in a language the patient can understand, the consent must be obtained by a person qualified to make the explanation.

For example, you are an intern who has consulted surgery to place a subclavian central venous line. You only know access must be obtained. You do not know why the internal jugular approach is not being used. On the phone the surgical resident says, "Can you go get the consent while I am coming up?" What should you do?

You must not be in a position to explain the risks of procedures that you did not decide on. If the patient develops a pneumothorax and you do not know why the internal jugular approach is not being used, you cannot adequately inform the patient. You are not certain why central access is being obtained at all. You must, at the risk of seeming difficult, tell the surgical resident that he must obtain the consent himself. If a complication occurs, you cannot say, "I was just getting a paper signed; I didn't know what it meant."

The same is true for a patient who signs consent. If you tell the patient that he could have a pneumothorax and might need a chest tube and document this, and the patient still signs consent, then you are not at risk. The patient also cannot say later, "I was just signing a piece of paper. I didn't know what it meant."

TELEPHONE CONSENT IS VALID

Consent obtained by a family member, health-care proxy, or other valid surrogate decision maker is valid even if obtained over the phone. This is a legitimate form of consent by an authorized surrogate decision maker.

> *For example,* a 65-year-old man is admitted to the hospital for a seizure. The head CT shows a ring or contrast-enhancing lesion consistent with a brain abscess. The patient remains persistently confused, but is not deteriorating. You need to perform a brain biopsy but there is no family member or health-care proxy who comes to visit him. His wife is housebound from multiple sclerosis and cannot get to the hospital. You have her on the phone but the nurse is refusing to be the witness for the consent, saying that telephone consent is not valid. What should you do?

As with all forms of verbal communication, oral advance directives, and telephone consent are more difficult to prove if contested. However, they are equally valid. If a health-care worker is uncomfortable taking the telephone consent, use another member of the health-care team to act as your witness for the consent. You can educate the nurse later. You can take consent for cardiothoracic surgery over the phone if that is the only way to speak to the surrogate.

The real questions about telephone consent are these:

1. Is the person you are speaking to really the surrogate?
2. Does the person know the patient's wishes?
3. Did you get the oral/telephone consent witnessed by another person so that the person giving consent cannot later deny having given consent?

PREGNANT WOMEN CAN REFUSE THERAPY

The prevailing consensus holds that a fetus is not a 'person' until birth. Hence, no matter what your personal feeling may be, the fetus does not have any intrinsic 'rights' as a person. So, even though a 34-week-old fetus would be a viable child if the fetus were removed from the uterus, all health-care decision making and ethics are based on the choices of the mother and her interests. If parents have a child born at 34 weeks of gestational age in need of a blood transfusion to save its life, they cannot refuse lifesaving therapy for the child even if they are Jehovah's Witnesses. The state would intervene in the interests of the child. However, if the same child at 34 weeks of gestational age is still in the uterus, the mother can refuse or accept whatever therapy she wishes without specific regard for the fetus. Hence, a pregnant woman may refuse a lifesaving transfusion. She may refuse a Caesarian section to remove the child even if this will put the life of the fetus at risk.

For any question concerning reproductive rights, decisions are based entirely on maternal wishes. The father has no legal right to make an informed consent for any pregnancy-related issue because the questions concern the body of the mother. A mother's autonomy over her own body is felt to be more important than the rights of the fetus or of the father. Only the mother can sign informed consent for any procedure or treatment during pregnancy. Any answer choice that has "Ask the father…" in it will always be wrong in terms of consent issues during pregnancy.

INFORMED CONSENT FOR A NEVER-COMPETENT PERSON

This is one of the most difficult subjects in ethics because the standard of this management has significantly evolved over the last several years. If the patient has Down syndrome and has a family member to make decisions for her then the question will be straightforward—ask for the consent of the parent or guardian. If there is no parent or guardian, the circumstance is much more difficult. A third-party court designee must make a decision based on the best interests of the patient even though the patient may never have expressed her feelings before.

The best way to obtain consent for a person who has lost the capacity to make decisions for him/herself is a health-care proxy or durable power of attorney. This is an advance directive (written or formal). An advance directive cannot even be given by a patient who has never had capacity. The same is true of a living will. The next best method of giving consent is "substituted judgment." In this case a person who knows the patient well tries to determine what decision she would make for herself if she were awake. This is also not possible for a person who has never been competent. The weakest form of consent is to act

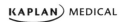

in the "best interests" of the patient. This is the weakest method of giving consent because it is filled with subjectivity and imprecision. However, it is the best method of obtaining consent for doctors treating a person who has never had capacity. A legal guardian which could be a family member must make the decision on behalf of the patient. In the absence of a family member the guardian is either appointed by the courts or is the administrator of the health-care facility, such as the medical director.

Chapter 4: **Confidentiality and Medical Records**

CONFIDENTIALITY

Physicians have a strong professional mandate to maintain the confidentiality of patients. Communications between patient and physician are highly privileged and this confidentiality can only be violated when there is potential harm to a third party or if there is a court order demanding the information. Medical information cannot be passed to anyone without the direct consent of the patient. Confidentiality also includes keeping a patient's medical information private even from his friends and family unless the patient expressly says it is okay to release the information. The fact that a patient may have a good relationship with his family and friends is absolutely no excuse to assume that the patient wants his medical information passed on to them. I have an excellent relationship with my mother; however, even though I am a doctor (or maybe because of it) she does not want me to know her list of medications. She has no obligation to give me a reason why she does not want me to know which medications she is taking. If I call her doctor and say, "I just want to help mom with her meds. What is she on?" Her physician is supposed to respond, "I'm sorry, but your mother hasn't authorized me to give you that information. I know you mean well, but I just can't talk to you about your mother's medical problems."

> *For example,* a 42-year-old man is hospitalized with chest pain. The patient is awake and alert. His wife comes to you demanding information about the patient, saying that she is his wife. She shows her identification card verifying this. What should you tell her?

You cannot release medical information to anyone about a patient unless the patient gives you permission to do so. Although it may seem rude and unreasonable, you must tell the patient's family members that you must ask your patient for permission before you can release his medical information.

> *For example,* the wife becomes infuriated and storms off the floor, threatening to sue you. You apologize to the patient for upsetting his wife by not speaking with her about his private medical problems. The patient responds "On the contrary, Doctor, you did great. Although she is still my wife, we are finalizing our divorce and we do not live together. I expect to be divorced and remarried within the next few months. She only wanted information about me to use against me in the divorce proceeding. Thanks for protecting my confidentiality."

RELEASE OF INFORMATION

Information transfer between physicians involved in the care of patients is a common occurrence. However, the information can only be transferred if the patient has signed a consent or release form requesting the transfer of information. It is the patient who must sign the consent to release the information, not the health-care provider. This is how the system guarantees that the patient's medically privileged information only transfers to those people to whom the patient wants it to go.

> *For example,* you receive a phone call from another physician who is well known to you in your local community. The physician says that one of your former patients has transferred his care to him and he is asking for a copy of the patient's medical record. What do you tell him?

You should tell another physician requesting information to send you the patient's signed release form before you send him the information.

GIVE MEDICAL INFORMATION TO THE
PATIENT FIRST, NOT THE FAMILY

For example, your patient is awaiting the results of a biopsy to tell whether or not she has cancer. Her son calls you and asks you to give him the information because the family is concerned that the bad news will depress his mother. He is sincere and genuine in his concern. What do you tell him?

Medical information such as the result of a biopsy must go to the patient first. There is no basis for informing the family and not the patient. It is exactly the opposite: without direct instruction from the patient, the family should not receive the patient's confidential medical information. Maybe the patient wants her family to know and maybe she doesn't. It is always the patient's decision. There is a rare exception in the case of a patient with a psychiatric disturbance in whom to inform if a medical condition might induce a suicide attempt.

RELEASE OF INFORMATION TO GOVERNMENTAL
ORGANIZATIONS AND THE COURTS

For example, an investigator from a local law enforcement agency comes to your office. He shows you proper identification stating that he is a government employee. He is looking for your patient's immigration status and for his medical condition. What do you tell the investigator?

If a member of a law enforcement agency comes to you with a subpoena or a court order that constitutes a search warrant then you must furnish him with the information that he requests. If the investigator does not have a search warrant, then you must refuse him access to the files. You are not under any obligation to make immigration status investigations of your patients nor to provide this information to third parties unless it is at the request of the patient. This right of privacy also covers genetic information. You must keep the medical information private from a patient's co-workers as well.

BREAKING CONFIDENTIALITY TO PREVENT HARM TO OTHERS

The right of a patient to privacy is not absolute. There are some exceptions as to when confidentiality can be broken in order to protect others. The Tarasof case (1976), in which a mentally ill patient told the psychiatrist of his intent to harm someone, is a famous example of this. In this type of case, the physician must inform law enforcement as well as the potential victim. Confidentiality is only broken in this way to prevent harm to others; this is rarely done.

Other cases in which it is lawful to break confidentiality include partner notification for sexually transmitted diseases such as syphilis and HIV. The patient's right to confidentiality in such cases is less important than another person's right to safety. However, all efforts must first be made to enlist the patient to inform the intimate partner. No lawsuit against a physician for breaking confidentiality in order to notify an innocent third party that his health may be at risk has been successful.

MEDICAL RECORDS

The physician or health-care facility physically owns the medical record, but the information contained within it is the property of the patient. Although the medical record as a physical object remains always in the hands of the health-care facility, the patient has an absolute right to free access to the information it contains. The information contained within a patient's medical record is covered by all the same rules of confidentiality as any other privileged medical information. You cannot release the medical record without the consent of the patient. No one except those directly involved in the care of the patient has a right to access to the record. Patients cannot take sole possession of the physical medical record but they have a right to access or copy the information.

> *For example,* you have a new patient with a complex history who has been trying to get a copy of her record from her previous doctor. The other practice said she must provide them with a valid reason for why she needs the chart. You call the other doctor's office trying to get the chart. The practice administrator informs you that the patient is extremely unpleasant and difficult. In addition, because the patient has not paid her bill the prior practice feels no obligation to provide you with the chart. The patient returns to see you the following day and asks what has become of her record. What do you tell her?

The patient has a right to her medical records. No one has a right to interfere with this for any reason. You should tell her that she should be allowed a copy of the chart. A patient does not have to give her doctor a reason for requesting her own property, and she is entitled to this information whether or not she is "pleasant." Furthermore, the medical record should not be "held hostage" to compel a patient to pay her medical bills. The need for information to take care of patients outweighs the physician's right to payment.

CORRECTING MEDICAL RECORD ERRORS

When an error in a chart needs correcting the doctor should draw a line through it and then initial the correction. This allows anyone reading the chart to see what was originally there and it ensures that medical errors are not being covered up. You cannot just remove pages from the chart or cover them over with correction fluid if there are mistakes. This makes it look as if you are hiding medical errors. If you forget to put in a note or document something and want to add it the next day, you cannot put a note in the chart with the old date. If you forgot to put a note in the chart documenting a patient's condition yesterday, you cannot write a note today with yesterday's date on it. In other words, you cannot 'back-date' notes. Your notes must always bear the current date and time.

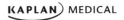

Chapter 5: **End-of-Life Issues**

WITHHOLDING AND WITHDRAWAL OF MEDICAL TREATMENT

Every competent adult with the capacity to understand his own medical problems has the right to determine what treatments he does or does not wish to receive. There is no ethical or legal distinction between withholding and withdrawal of medical treatment.

> *For example,* a 60-year-old man with diabetes and hypertension develops renal insufficiency to the point of needing dialysis. He is equivocal about spending the rest of his life on dialysis, but he agrees to start. The patient is not depressed and is fully alert. Six months after starting dialysis, he comes to realize very clearly that he absolutely does not wish to continue. You have no doubt that the patient has full capacity to understand the implications of this decision. What should you do?

Although there may be an emotional distinction between withholding dialysis and stopping it after it has started, there is no ethical distinction between the two. If I don't like to play basketball there is no legal distinction between my never starting to play basketball or playing a few games and then not doing it anymore. It is my right to stop. If I hire you to repair my house, but after a few days I decide that I don't like the work you are doing, I have the right to tell you to stop working on my house. You cannot say, "Sorry, once we start a job we finish it whether the owner likes it or not." I have the right to refuse to allow you to work on my house and the right to tell you to stop after you started. The patient has the right to stop treatment.

> *For example,* an elderly man with COPD progresses to the point of needing mechanical ventilation on a chronic basis. He tells you, after long consideration, that he just does not want to live on a ventilator. What should you tell him?

You must honor his wishes. This patient is an adult with the capacity to understand his medical problems, so he has the right to choose whether or not he wishes to be on a ventilator. The wrong answers include getting a court order, treating him against his will, and asking the family for consent.

> *For example,* a 42-year-old man sustains a cervical spine injury at C1 and C2 leaving him paralyzed from the neck down and ventilator dependent. He is very upbeat and cheerful. He says he will get better and wants to be maintained permanently on the ventilator. You clearly inform him that he is wrong and he will never improve. He says he wants the ventilator forever, or until he is cured. What do you tell him?

Once again, you must honor his wishes. This is an adult patient with the capacity to understand his medical condition. Although you may disagree with his judgment about the likelihood of his recovery, he has every right to try. Unreasonable optimism is not the equivalent of incompetence. Overall, this case will be the easiest to agree with, because most ethical dilemmas do not involve a conscious patient wishing to continue care, but rather involve patients who have lost capacity and the dilemma of whether or not to withdraw treatment.

> *For example,* a woman with aplastic anemia becomes transfusion dependent. After a few months she becomes tired of it and refuses all subsequent transfusions. She has the capacity to understand that she will die without the transfusion, although she is not suicidal. What do you tell her?

You must honor her wishes. She is an adult with the capacity to understand her medical problems. The consequences of refusing therapy have been explained to her. It would be incorrect to advise her to get a psychiatric consultation, to obtain a court order compelling her to accept the transfusion, to ask the family to authorize the procedure, or to ask for an ethics committee evaluation. Psychiatric consultation is only necessary if the patient's capacity to understand is uncertain. If the patient is clearly lucid and not depressed, no psychiatric evaluation is necessary.

> *For example,* an HIV-positive Jehovah's Witness who is now pregnant needs a transfusion to live and have a healthy baby. She categorically refuses. She is not depressed and is fully alert. What do you tell her?

You must honor her wishes. You cannot transfuse a competent adult against her will. The situation would be different if the patient were a minor in which case the doctor would be compelled to transfuse. The fact that the patient is pregnant does not alter the answer. The prevailing consensus is that personhood begins after birth. Until delivered, the fetus is considered another part of the mother's body. The wrong answers will include getting a court order or asking the father of the child for consent. Another wrong answer would be waiting until the patient is no longer conscious and then transfusing her.

The answers to all of the examples described in this section are clear because in each case the patient is an adult with the capacity to understand his or her medical problems. If the case describes depression in the patient then you should choose psychiatric consultation, or choose a trial of either behavioral therapy or antidepressant medication as the answer.

Patients have the right to try therapy for a while and then stop it if it does not suit them. This is true even if it means they will die from stopping dialysis, mechanical ventilation, HIV medications, or blood transfusions. The type of treatment does not change the answer. A CBC or cardiac bypass is ethically and legally indistinguishable. Treating a patient without consent is legally equivalent to assault and battery or any other form of unwanted touching. Therefore, in a sense, treating a patient against his will and without his consent is like mugging the patient or beating him up.

There is no distinction between withholding and withdrawing care. If you are doing something the patient does not want, you cannot say, "Well, sorry, but I already started, and I really have to continue."

ADVANCE DIRECTIVES

Definition

An advance directive is the method by which a patient communicates his wishes for his health care in advance of becoming unable to make decisions for himself. The advance directive is a by-product of the success of medical therapies such as the mechanical ventilator that can keep a patient alive when in the past he would have died. Because of these therapies, doctors are now in the position of trying to determine what each patient wanted for himself in terms of his health care. The advance directive is part of the concept of autonomy. The advance directive tells the physician what the patient's wishes are so that the less accurate forms of decision making, such as substituted judgment or making a decision based on another person's idea of the best interests of the patient, become avoidable.

Health-Care Proxy

The two most common forms of advance directives are the living will and the health-care proxy. The health-care proxy or "medical power of attorney" is the durable power of attorney for health-care decisions or medical proxy. The concept of a "durable" power of attorney is critical because the word "durable" means it remains in effect even after the patient loses decision-making capacity because of medical illness. Other forms of legal proxies, such as a financial proxy, become ineffective after the patient loses consciousness. The health-care proxy is a person chosen specifically by the patient to make health-care decisions for her in the event that she cannot make decisions for herself. These decisions are limited to health care, not finance. Advance directive documents may also have written instructions to give boundaries to care. For example, a patient may want to receive antibiotics, but not want to receive chemotherapy or dialysis. However, the main focus of the proxy is to designate a person or "agent" who speaks to the physician regarding consent issues for all treatments and tests, as well as discusses issues of withdrawing and withholding treatment. The proxy speaks for the patient. Because the patient chooses the proxy as her representative, the proxy overrules all other decision makers. There is a strong presumption that the proxy knows the patient's wishes. The proxy is not there to give his personal opinion as to what he thinks should be done for the patient. The proxy is there to communicate the patient's original wishes in order to ensure that they are carried out.

The proxy is like a messenger. The patient writes the message—her wishes for her own health care—and the proxy delivers the message. You would not want your proxy to alter your wishes any more than you would want your mailman to rewrite your letters.

The proxy is also like a waiter. The patient tells the waiter what kind of food he wants to eat (what kind of medicines and tests he wants). The proxy places the order in the kitchen. The proxy is not there to alter your expressed wishes. You would not want to order chicken and have the waiter tell the kitchen you want fish. Your waiter tries to understand what you want to eat. The waiter doesn't walk up and tell you, "You look weak and anemic. You are having a rare steak tonight, which is what is best for you." Now the main difference is that this is a "restaurant" in which the customer is unconscious and can't tell you exactly what he wants.

The proxy makes decisions based on two parameters:

1. The patient's directly expressed health-care wishes
2. What the patient would have wanted if he/she had capacity

These are the two overriding principles:

1. The health-care proxy must carry out the written and verbal wishes expressed to him regarding the patient's health care; the basis for which is sometimes just his understanding of what the patient would want if she were awake to make the decision.

2. The proxy outweighs all other potential decision makers, including the family.

For example, a 75-year-old man arrives at the emergency department febrile, short of breath, and confused. Many family members accompany the patient, including his wife, his siblings, his children, and his grandchildren. The physician wants to perform an emergency lumbar puncture, which the patient's wife and siblings are refusing. His 25-year-old granddaughter walks up with a health-care proxy form signed by the patient designating her as the proxy. She insists that you do the lumbar puncture stating that was her understanding of the patient's wishes. The rest of the family, including the wife, refuses the lumbar puncture stating that they know the patient's wishes better. What do you do?

Legally, you should honor the health-care proxy above all other decision makers, regardless of the level of closeness in biological relationship or frequency of contact. You cannot tell who in a family knows the patients wishes best unless the patient is awake to tell you. The proxy designation is the patient's way of telling you who he feels will represent his wishes.

In the absence of an advance directive there is a list of relative importance in terms of surrogate decision makers. You should start first with the spouse, then parents, then adult children, then siblings, then friends. This is an approximation only. If the family is split in its wishes there is no easy solution. When the family is split and there is no proxy, you must refer to the ethics committee or the courts for a judgment.

Living Will

A living will is a written form of advance directive that outlines the care that a patient would want for herself if she were to lose the ability to communicate or the capacity to understand her medical problems. The etiology of the loss of decision-making capacity is irrelevant.

A living will can range from being an extremely precise document outlining the exact types of care that a patient wants or does not want all the way to being a vague, useless document that makes nonspecific statements such as "no heroic care." The main problem with the living will is that most of the time it lacks precision because the patient does not explicitly state which tests and treatments she wants for herself. A document saying "no extraordinary care" is virtually worthless. What does "extraordinary care" mean? Does that mean a ventilator or chemotherapy, or dialysis, or blood tests, or all of them, or none of them? If the living will is explicit in listing the precise names of the tests and treatments that the patient would like to receive (or not to receive), then it is useful. For instance, a living will that says "No intubation, no cardiopulmonary resuscitation, no dialysis, and no blood transfusions" is very useful and allows for easy following.

> *For example,* a 78-year-old woman is admitted with metastatic cancer leading to a change in mental status secondary to hypercalcemia. She has a living will in her record that states, "In the event that I become unable to speak for myself for any reason I wish to express my wish that I not be intubated or placed on a ventilator under any circumstances. I also do not wish to receive dialysis. Blood testing and antibiotics are acceptable." What should you do?

The living will is most valid and usable when specific tests and treatments are outlined. In the case above, follow the direction of the living will and carry out the patient's wishes. A living will would overrule the wishes of the family because the living will communicates the patient's own wishes. As a matter of autonomy, the patient's clearly expressed wishes always take precedence over the wishes of other decision makers, such as family members.

The major issue with the use of a living will is that it is very difficult, in advance of the illness, to be certain which medical treatments and tests will be necessary. It is very difficult for a layperson to say, "I do not want an albumin infusion with my large volume paracentesis," or "A biopsy for diagnostic purposes by interventional radiology is acceptable, but I do not want an open biopsy in the operating room," or "I agree to antibiotics, but not to amphotericin." A health-care proxy allows for far greater flexibility. However, if a patient really does write out the specific names of the most common treatments and the parameters for their use, then the living will can be a very useful document.

No Capacity and No Advance Directives

Here is what is very clear about withholding and withdrawal of care decisions:

- An adult with capacity can decide to accept or refuse any therapy offered.
- An adult without capacity can be managed with a health-care proxy or a living will if the living will is sufficiently clear and specific enough.

Unfortunately, the vast majority of patients, even at older age and with life-threatening illnesses, do not have a formal advance directive. Decision making can be much more difficult in this circumstance. If the family is united and in agreement, then there is no difficulty with making decisions for the patient. The main issue again comes to demonstrating the best evidence of knowing the patient's wishes.

> *For example,* a 64-year-old man suffers a severe intracranial bleed leaving him comatose and paralyzed. His wife, sister, and four children are in the hospital. They come to see you because they are unanimously asking that you remove the endotracheal tube and leave the patient to die. The patient repeatedly made this wish known to his family. What should you do?

For a patient without the capacity to understand his medical problems and no health-care proxy or living will, the path of management is clear as long as all of the family members are in agreement. You can remove the endotracheal tube and let the patient die if everyone says that is what the patient has said he wanted. The endotracheal tube is a medical therapy like any other. The patient has the right to refuse it. The patient's family or others who know the patient well can provide the patient's previously expressed wishes—an oral advanced directive.

> *For example,* a 78-year-old woman has been admitted to a nursing home with advanced dementia. She has difficulty maintaining oral intake sufficient to survive. The nursing home wants to place a nasogastric tube for feeding. The husband and the son expressly state that the patient said she "never wanted to be maintained like a vegetable" and "I don't want to be put on a ventilator or have a feeding tube down my throat." What should you do?

Are the family members passing on information about what the patient said, or are they telling you to do what they think is best for the patient? You can do virtually anything in the care of a patient, even without an advance directive, as long as the family is united in passing on what the patient said she wanted for her own care. Problems arise when the family is in disagreement about what the patient said or when. Instead of expressing the patient's wishes, they are representing what they want for the patient. Having a family member express a patient's wishes is equivalent to having him cast a vote on the patient's behalf. If a person cannot speak, another person can mail in her vote for her if she has clearly told this person which candidate she wants to vote for. If she told her brother that wanted to vote republican and he sends in her ballot stating this, then he is acting on her wishes as her agent. On the other hand, if he believes she would prefer to vote democrat if she were awake or he believes one candidate is better for her then this represents a much lower level of evidence for her vote. Likewise, if he knows what she wants because she told him, then he can stop the ventilator, the blood testing, the chemotherapy, the dialysis, or any other treatment.

Ethics Committee and Referral to the Courts

When there is no clear advance directive and the family does not agree on what the patient wanted for himself or herself, then the right answer is to refer to the ethics committee and finally the courts.

Here is a list of the various kinds of consent, with the most desirable listed first:

- Direct patient wish verbalized by the patient
- Formal advance directive such as a proxy or a living will
- Oral advance directive
- United group of family and friends
- Group of family members disagreeing on what the patient would have wanted

In cases where there is no living will or proxy and the family members are not in agreement, the next step is to "encourage consensus," "request discussion," or "talk with the parties involved." If consensus is not possible, you should refer the case to the hospital ethics committee. The last step to pursue in the absence of a clear consensus is referral to the courts or "seek judicial intervention."

For example, the Terry Schiavo case ended up in the courts because her husband and several of her friends said the patient told them that she never wanted to be maintained in a persistent vegetative state. The patient's parents stated that she never said that. The ethics committee does not have direct legal power and their decisions are not always universally binding. If the ethics committee is unable to build consensus, or the involved parties ignore the ethics committee, then judicial intervention is necessary.

"DO NOT RESUSCITATE" (DNR) ORDERS

A "Do Not Resuscitate" (DNR) order means if the patient dies, i.e., has cardiopulmonary arrest, the doctor does not perform chest compressions, attempt electrical cardioversion, or administer acute anti-arrhythmic medications. That is all, nothing more. Death of the patient in this case means the sudden loss of pulse, blood pressure, and the ability to breathe.

> *For example,* a 42-year-old HIV-positive man is admitted for hematuria that is most likely from kidney cancer. He is DNR. Urology is consulted and they think a kidney biopsy is in order as well as a possible nephrectomy, however, they do not want to do either one because the "patient is DNR and therefore preterminal." What should you tell them?

The most common misunderstanding about DNR orders is that being DNR must mean the patient is preterminal and just about to die. Another common misunderstanding is that a person who is DNR should not get other aspects of routine good care such as surgery, biopsies, or dialysis. DNR is not a stamp of certain death. If the patient has renal cell carcinoma and needs a biopsy and nephrectomy, then the decision to do these procedures has to do with the patient's medical needs and complications and not the DNR. DNR just means that the physician should take cardiopulmonary arrest as the end-point of therapy. Usually when a patient dies there is a sudden, rapid upgrade in the amount of therapy, such as giving intravenous medications, chest compressions, and electrical cardioversion. A patient may still undergo surgery or be placed in the intensive care unit if he is DNR.

When patients have cardiopulmonary arrest, there is presumed consent to cardiopulmonary resuscitation unless the patient specifically and expressively refused this therapy in advance.

> *For example,* a 42-year-old man with AIDS is being taken to the operating room for a nephrectomy. The surgical resident shrugs his shoulders and says, "Oh well, at least we can move fast. The DNR means it doesn't really matter if the surgery is successful, so the DNR is kind of a relief." What should you tell him?

DNR does not mean patients should receive less of anything except cardiopulmonary resuscitation. DNR is not a "get-out-of-jail-free" card, which absolves physicians of wrongdoing or serves as an excuse for making a mistake. DNR does not mean it is okay just to let the patient die, or that the doctor does not have to be as careful. A patient can still be intubated and maintained on a ventilator if she is DNR. This is a confusing point because endotracheal intubation is often a part of the normal resuscitative process. If the patient is DNR and he loses his pulse then the doctor would not intubate because the intubation here would be considered part of the 'Code' or resuscitative/CPR management. However, if the patient remains alive and has advancing lung disease, the patient can still be intubated. In this case, the doctor would only defer CPR if the patient were DNR. Doctors do not have to remove the endotracheal tube of all patients who choose to be DNR. Many patients will not allow themselves to be made DNR because they believe the medical staff will not be as aggressive in their other treatments.

> *For example,* a 68-year-old man with basal cell cancer is admitted for evaluation and treatment of a fever. He has been DNR for the last six months. After the chest X ray, urinalysis, and blood culture are done he still has a fever of unknown etiology. When you ask the resident why he hasn't done more tests, the response is, "Well, we will get to it, but there isn't much of a rush, after all, the patient is DNR." What do you tell him?

DNR does not mean anything more than deferring CPR, such as chest compressions and electrical cardioversion. In this case, it would also eliminate endotracheal intubation if this treatment were part of the resuscitative effort. That is all. The doctor is expected to manage pain and the diagnosis of other medical problems just as aggressively as she would in a non-DNR patient unless the patient has specifically chosen to defer those other forms of therapy. Doctors do not automatically have to have the DNR order reversed just to be in the intensive care unit or to go to surgery.

FLUIDS AND NUTRITION ISSUES

Adults with the Capacity to Understand

The artificial administration of fluids and nutrition is a medical procedure and treatment that can be accepted or refused by a competent adult in exactly the same manner as any other treatment. "Artificial administration" basically refers to any form of nutrition other than eating. "Artificial" specifically means feedings or fluids administered by nasogastric, gastric, or jejunostomy tube placement. "Artificial nutrition" would also refer to intravenously administered nutrition such as total parenteral nutrition (TPN), also referred to as hyperalimentation.

> *For example,* a 47-year-old theoretical physicist with amyotrophic lateral sclerosis has become progressively more disabled to the point of being virtually immobile in a wheelchair. He is unable to work in a meaningful way. He has pulled out the gastric feeding tube and refuses to allow its reinsertion. His wife, who is also his nurse, is insisting that you reinsert it. What should you tell her?

Forcible insertion by anyone of an artificial feeding device into an adult patient with the capacity to understand the meaning of its removal is not allowed. If the patient's wishes are clearly expressed, this is the same as refusing a ventilator, blood testing, or dialysis. This refusal is subject to the same criteria as the refusal of other therapies. You must be sure there isn't a severe depression underlying the refusal and that the patient understands that he may die without the tube. If there is no depression, then the patient has the right to refuse a therapy even if he will die without it. Putting the tube back into a person who has refused it is considered the same as assault and battery.

Adults Who Have Lost the Capacity to Understand

Deciding what to do about artificial nutrition when the patient cannot speak for herself is a much harder circumstance. Nutrition is the single most difficult issue in terms of withholding and withdrawing treatment. We can never withhold ordinary nutrition like food to eat and water to drink. The standard of certainty regarding a patient's wishes in terms of artificial nutrition is much higher than with other therapies. We must have very clear evidence of what the patient's wishes were in regard to artificial nutrition.

If there is a health-care proxy, and the healthcare agent says, "The patient clearly told me that they didn't want tube feeds," you may withhold the therapy. If there is a living will where the patient themselves wrote, "I do not wish to have a nasogastric tube or other forms of artificial nutrition," you may withhold the therapy. If there is no advance directive, but the family is in uniform agreement that the patient had expressed the wish never to have tube feeds, you may withhold the therapy. If clear wishes regarding fluids and nutrition were never clearly expressed, then there is implied consent for the feeding based on the presumption that it would be the patient's wish to be fed and on the fact that feeding and hydration are in the patient's best interest.

Emotionally, the standard is different from the standard used to determine whether or not ordinary testing such as blood tests or CT scans should be done. The proxy and family can say, "The patient never specifically told me that he would not want a liver biopsy or MRI of the brain, but my understanding of his wishes in general is that he doesn't want to undergo these procedures." This would not be the same for nutrition. Decisions on withholding and withdrawing of artificial fluids and nutrition should be treated the same way as any other medical treatment. There is a higher standard of evidence for decision making in some states. That is why this issue is so complex. Few people have left a specific, written document concerning their desire for tube feeding.

The evidence has to be clear that a patient does not want artificial nutrition. The routine assumption is that most people wish to be fed as a part of ordinary care. If the evidence is not clear, then a referral to an ethics committee, or possibly to the courts, is necessary. The level of evidence regarding the patient's wishes necessary for withholding and withdrawing artificial nutrition has been treated by some courts as the same as the level of evidence required in a criminal case. The system errs on the side of caution—perhaps letting a few guilty people go free rather than sending a single innocent person to jail or execution. If you lost consciousness suddenly and left no specific instructions, wouldn't you want there to be a need for convincing evidence that you didn't want to be fed before your relatives were able to withhold nutrition and possibly let you die? Ethical consensus holds that decisions to provide or forgo artificial nutrition and hydration (ANH) for patients who lack capacity should be made according to the same standards as those used for any other medical treatment. Despite this consensus, certain states impose more stringent standards for withholding or withdrawal of ANH compared to other medical treatments.

PHYSICIAN-ASSISTED SUICIDE

In physician-assisted suicide, the physician provides the patient with the means of ending his own life. The doctor does not actually administer the substance that ends the patient's life. Although there is national controversy on the issue, the answer on the USMLE is very clear; physician-assisted suicide is always considered incorrect and ethically unacceptable. This is true even if there is a local state law permitting the procedure. What is legal does not automatically equal what is ethical. Generally, physician-assisted suicide is requested by patients who have a terminal disease and a limited life expectancy anyway. Nevertheless, the severity of the disease and even the discomfort and suffering of the patient do not change the answer. Physician-assisted suicide is always considered to be wrong on the USMLE. The primary issue is one of intent. Physician-assisted suicide is inimical, or absolutely contrary, to the role of the physician to save life. This is true even if the patient is requesting the assistance. A physician cannot ethically honor a patient's wishes to be provided with the means to end his life.

EUTHANASIA

With euthanasia the physician goes even further in ending a patient's life than in physician-assisted suicide. Euthanasia actually means that the health-care worker is prescribing and administering the method of death. There is no place in the United States where euthanasia is legal. A physician cannot legally administer a lethal injection or any other form of therapy that will help end life. This is true even if the patient is preterminal. Euthanasia is ethically unacceptable.

TERMINAL SEDATION OF THE "LAW OF DOUBLE EFFECT"

There is an enormous difference between administering a lethal injection and giving pain medications that might inadvertently shorten a patient's life. The issue is one of intent. If the intent is to end life, it is wrong. If the intent is to relieve suffering and accidentally—as an unintended effect—the patient's life is shortened, then the treatment is acceptable. This is comparable to the difference between a charitable donation and being robbed. If I give $1,000 to charity to help others it is a virtue. If I steal even one dollar from you, it is a crime. Both events result in the transfer of money, however, the ethical distinction is enormous.

For example, a 67-year-old man is admitted with metastatic prostate cancer to the bones. He is in excruciating pain despite your present treatment. He has a history of COPD and the house staff are concerned that increasing his pain medications will decrease his respiratory drive. What should you do?

As long as you are not purposely giving high-dose opiates in order to end the patient's life, it is acceptable to give the pain medications even if it might decrease his respiratory drive. The primary ethical duty is to relieve suffering. You cannot just leave the patient to suffer. Give the patient the amount of medication they need to relieve the pain even if, unintentionally, there is an adverse effect on the respiratory drive.

FUTILE CARE

The physician is not under an obligation to give treatment or perform tests that will not benefit the patient. This is true even if the patient or the family is demanding it. The major problem in withholding or withdrawing therapy on the basis of it being futile is being sure that there will be no benefit. It is hard always to be certain if the treatment will not help. If it is clear that there will be no benefit then you should not give it.

For example, a 57-year-old woman with cryptogenic cirrhosis is under your care. She is septic and has severe variceal bleeding as well as encephalopathy not responding to lactulose. She is hypotensive and on pressors as well as intubated from respiratory failure and you expect her to die from her liver disease in the next few days. She develops Hepatorenal syndrome and has developed uremia. The family is requesting placement of a fistula for dialysis. What should you tell them?

In this case, there is a clear underlying preterminal condition. You should not start dialysis or place the fistula. Dialysis in this case will not change the outcome. Dialysis in this case would not prolong meaningful life. Because in this case dialysis would only prolong the dying process, withholding it is ethical, even if the family is requesting it.

DETERMINATION OF DEATH AND BRAIN DEATH

The two methods of defining death are termination of heartbeat and brain death. If the heart is still beating, but the patient is brain dead, then the person is dead. Brain-death criteria have enormous significance for the ability to harvest organs for donation as well as in criminal cases.

For example, a man is arrested for armed robbery in which he assaults another man. The victim has sustained cerebral herniation and has lost all spontaneous respirations, cognitive function, and brainstem reflexes. You are called as an expert witness to advise the court. The alleged assailant's defense lawyer tells the judge that the charge on his client should only be assault and battery, not murder, because the patient's heart is still beating. The defense lawyer contends that the victim can be alive for many years in this condition. The maximum penalty in some states for murder is life imprisonment or execution. The penalty for assault may be only 10 to 20 years in prison. What should you tell the judge?

Brain death is the legal definition of death. An assault leading to brain death is a murder. Brain death is irreversible and permanent. A beating heart that maintains blood pressure and pulse does not equal being alive. When we, as physicians, determine the criteria for brain death are present, this is the legally accepted standard of death.

Brain death is a loss of brainstem reflexes such as:

- Pupilary light reflex
- Corneal reflexes
- Oculocephalic (doll's eyes) reflexes
- Caloric responses to iced water stimulation of the tympanic membrane
- The absence of spontaneous respirations

You can determine loss of respirations by removing the ventilator and observing for signs of respiration. If the criteria for brain death are met, then an EEG or cerebral blood-flow study are not necessary. In other words, the clinical criteria of the absence of breathing and brainstem reflexes are more important than an EEG. This is because EEG activity would be of limited meaning if a patient meets the clinical brain-death criteria.

Brain death should only be determined to be present if you have excluded other causes of markedly decreased brainstem and respiratory function. You must be certain that the patient is not suffering from an overdose of barbiturates, hypothermia, hypotension, or the use of neuromuscular blocking agents such as pancuronium, vecuronium, or succinylcholine. These can all simulate brain death.

For example, a 35-year-old woman is admitted after having a seizure at a party. Her head CT scan shows an intracranial bleed. She is intubated because of the loss of spontaneous respiration. There are no pupilary, corneal, oculocephalic, or cold caloric reflexes elicited. Which of the following should you do next?

a. EEG
b. EKG
c. Urine toxicology screen
d. Psychiatric evaluation
e. Ethics committee evaluation

This patient has met most of the criteria for brain death. An EKG is not necessary to diagnose death at any point. Auscultation of the heart is all that is required to document the stopping of the heart. You should exclude intoxication with CNS depressant drugs and hypothermia prior to determining that the patient is brain dead.

Brain death does not specifically require determination by a neurologist if the physician managing the patient is comfortable with the criteria described and how to verify them. This is similar to not needing a psychiatrist in order to determine capacity. If the patient is clearly not brain dead because their pupils are reactive or they have spontaneous breathing, a neurologist is unnecessary.

If the patient is brain dead, then they are dead. The physician does not need a court order or a relative's permission to remove life support. The doctor does not need to ask anyone's permission to stop the ventilator or other treatment, although USMLE will always want you to answer "discuss with the family," "explain your findings," or "build consensus" first rather than just turning off the ventilator. This may seem contradictory. You should always explain what brain death means to the patient's family. You need to answer "explain the meaning of brain death to the family" as the first choice if it appears.

On the other hand, the family's permission or consent is not required for terminating life support, because a person who is brain dead is considered dead. Insurance companies will not pay for the hospitalization or management of those patients who are dead. You can harvest organs for transplantation from a brain-dead person if the family consents. You do not have to wait for the person's heart to stop. Actually, it is preferable to remove the organs while the heart is still beating because the viability of the transplanted organ strongly correlates to how long it was unperfused after removal from the donor's body.

Chapter 6: **Reproductive Issues**

ABORTION

An adult woman has an unrestricted access to abortion through the end of the first trimester. First-trimester abortions are clearly unrestricted. Women do not need the approval or consent of anyone else to obtain a first-trimester abortion. In the second trimester the decision is still between a woman and her physician, but the ease of access to a second-trimester abortion is less clear. States may place regulations on free access to a second-trimester abortion. However, second-trimester abortions are preponderantly still performed at the patient's discretion. Third-trimester abortions are not freely available, because the fetus is potentially viable. Third-trimester abortions are clearly restricted. Consent by the father for an abortion is not required; the fetus is considered as a part of the woman's body and does not have the individual rights of 'personhood' until after birth.

There is no compulsion on the part of the physician to perform an abortion if performing this procedure is ethically unacceptable to the physician. The patient has a right to have an abortion, but they don't have a right to force you to do it, if it is objectionable to you.

In addition, it is considered unethical for a patient to seek an abortion for the purposes of gender selection. It is considered ethically unacceptable to determine the gender of the fetus and then abort the fetus if the sex in unacceptable to the patient.

> *For example,* a 23-year-old woman comes to your office seeking an abortion. You perform gynecologic procedures and you have been trained to do abortions in the past. However, you no longer find it morally acceptable to perform the procedure although you know how. The patient is insisting on having the abortion and is angry with you for "abandoning your patient." What should you tell her?

As a general rule, if there is a procedure that the patient wants but that you do not feel ethically comfortable performing, you should refer the patient to another physician. You cannot be compelled to accept a patient you do not want or to do a procedure with which you do not agree. The physician must voluntarily agree to the relationship.

CONTRACEPTION

There is no limitation on the access to contraception for either a man or a woman. It is entirely at the discretion of the patient. This is equally true for minors. Contraception is one of the issues for which a minor is considered partially emancipated. Parental consent is not necessary to obtain contraception.

STERILIZATION

Both women and men have free access to sterilization. Consent is only necessary from the patient. Spousal consent is not required for sterilization. All reproductive issues, including abortion, contraception, and sterilization can be performed over the objection of the spouse. Each person has autonomy over his or her own body.

MINORS

Parental consent is not necessary for either contraception or prenatal care. In cases involving reproductive issues for minors, the answer will be either to just treat the minor or to "encourage discussion" with the parents. Even though parental consent is not necessary, USMLE will still want you to encourage disclosure to parents about most reproductive issues involving minors. The rules on parental consent in the case of abortion are less clear. Some states require parental consent for abortions and others do not. Because USMLE is a national examination and the rules on parental consent for abortion vary from state to state, there cannot be a single answer that either says "no parental consent" or "yes, parental consent is necessary." Therefore, the answer will be "encourage the patient to discuss the issue with parents."

DONATION OF SPERM AND EGGS

There is no limitation on a patient's permissibility to donate sperm and unfertilized eggs. In addition, payment may be received for sperm and unfertilized egg donations. In other words, there is no legal or ethical contraindication to selling sperm and unfertilized eggs. There is, however, a prohibition against selling fertilized eggs. Fertilized eggs may be donated, but not sold.

Chapter 7: **Organ and Tissue Donation**

AUTONOMY OF THE DONOR

Organ and tissue donation is a voluntary event entirely at the discretion of the live donor. The principle of autonomy is fully in play here.

> *For example,* a 35-year-old-man is dying of hepatic failure. His brother is fully HLA matched and a highly compatible donor. There are no other donors at this time and the patient will likely not survive long enough to find another donor. You are screening the brother for the donation, but he is not willing to undergo the surgery for the partial donation. What should you do?

There is nothing you or anyone—including a court of law—can do to compel a person to donate an organ or tissue if he clearly chooses not to do so. The need of the recipient has no impact on mandating a donor to donate. This is true even if the donation is uncomplicated for the donor and the recipient will die without it.

ORGAN DONOR NETWORK ASKS FOR CONSENT FOR DONATION

> *For example,* a 30-year-old woman is your patient in the intensive care unit for respiratory failure. The patient has had a motor vehicle accident and has sustained a massive intracranial hemorrhage. The patient is brain dead and will be removed from the ventilator. You know that there are numerous patients in your hospital waiting for organs. The family of the patient is with you. You have an excellent relationship with the family and they trust you. What should you do about the donation?

Only the organ donor network or uniform network for organ sharing should obtain consent for an organ donation. The medical team taking care of the patient should not ask for the donation. Even if your relationship with the family is excellent, the organ donor network has an enormously greater success rate in obtaining consent. Physicians that ask for consent for organ donation are far more likely to be refused. Because a greater number of refusals would lead to a loss of potential organs for donation when the shortage of available organs is critical, it is against the law for doctors to obtain this consent. By legal statute, only those specifically trained to obtain consent for organ donation should approach the family for this consent.

In addition, there is the perception of an enormous conflict of interest on the part of the family when a caregiver attempts to obtain consent. When a caregiver asks for consent, it leads some families to believe that the health-care team is not doing everything possible to preserve the life of the patient. This makes it seem that the priority of the health-care team is to obtain organs. It is essential for the health-care team to preserve its relationship with the family as the advocates for preserving the life of the patient. In addition, the organ donation network has a much greater chance of obtaining consent, so if the primary health-care team tries to obtain consent, it could lead to a loss of needed organs.

PAYMENT FOR DONATIONS

With the exception of renewable tissues such as sperm, unfertilized eggs, and blood, payment for organs is considered ethically unacceptable. People must not be in the business of selling organs. The economic aspects of organ donation must be minimized so that people believe that the patients who need organs the most will get them, not that the wealthy will get preferential treatment. It is, however, acceptable to cover the cost to the donor of donation. There is a difference between reimbursing the donor for the cost of donation and creating a financial incentive for people to "sell" organs.

ORGAN DONOR CARDS

Although an organ donor card gives an indication of a patient's wishes for donation, family consent is still necessary for donation. Family objection can overrule the organ donor card.

Chapter 8: **Reportable Illnesses**

Physicians and laboratories are mandated to report a number of medical illnesses. The main purpose in reporting illnesses is both epidemiologic as well as to interrupt the spread of certain communicable diseases. The illnesses that are always reportable include AIDS, syphilis, tuberculosis, gonorrhea, and all of the childhood diseases such as measles, mumps, rubella, and pertussis. The list of other reportable diseases is extensive. These diseases are reportable by somebody, not necessarily the physician.

Physicians are always legally protected for participating in partner notification. In general, the health department performs the majority of contact-tracing events as well as notifying those that have been in close contact of the possibility of infection. The name of the source patient is always protected.

Partner notification exists for diseases such as HIV/AIDS, syphilis, gonorrhea, and tuberculosis. In addition, the health department can incarcerate patients with tuberculosis to prevent the spread of disease. If a patient won't tell his or her partner, then you must answer that you must follow your duty to report. If the source patient still won't tell his or her partner, you are within your legal right to tell the innocent third party. Partner notification and reportable illnesses are an example of one of the few times that the patient's autonomy can be superseded because of the necessity of protecting others. My right to autonomy ends where your safety begins. I have an absolute right to privacy, except when my restaurant serves food infected with salmonella, and then the patient's rights to autonomy become less important than protecting others from harm.

Tuberculosis has special reporting and public-health issues. In addition to doing contact tracing of the contacts in order to do PPD testing, there is the special issue of incarceration for tuberculosis. Patients with tuberculosis should be isolated for about two weeks, which is approximately the amount of time that is takes for sputum to become negative for acid-fast bacilli. If a patient refuses to take antituberculosis therapy, physicians have the option of

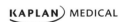

incarcerating the patient to prevent them from spreading the disease. This is only for those who still have positive stains of their sputum for acid-fast bacilli.

Incarceration for tuberculosis is not the same thing as being arrested. It has nothing to do with the criminal-justice system. The incarceration occurs in a hospital not in a prison or jail. You cannot force-feed tuberculosis medications, but you can prevent people from walking at their leisure in the community to spread disease. Incarceration is a last resort and is only used after all other options have been exhausted in terms of having discussions with the patient and offering directly observed therapy at home.

Chapter 9: **HIV-Related Issues**

CONFIDENTIALITY

As with all medical information there is a presumption of confidentiality on the part of the physician. Because of the social stigma of HIV there is an additional layer of confidentiality and consent required. When a patient enters the hospital or other health-care facility there is general consent given that allows the routine testing of blood for chemistry and hematology and so on. There is an additional HIV-related consent required to test for HIV. When a patient signs a release to distribute or transmit medical information there is an additional consent required for HIV or AIDS-related information. You cannot mandate automatic HIV testing of patients without their specific informed consent that you will be testing for HIV.

> *For example,* a woman comes at 10 weeks of pregnancy for prenatal care. She has a history of sexually transmitted diseases such as gonorrhea. You offer HIV testing, which the patient refuses, as a routine part of prenatal care. She returns at 14 and 18 weeks of pregnancy but is still refusing because of anxiety that she may be positive. You inform the patient that there are medications that can reduce transmission from mother to child to less than 2 percent. She persists in her refusal. What should you do now?

Although there are medications to prevent transmission of HIV to the fetus during pregnancy, you cannot compel mandatory testing of pregnant women. The woman has the right to refuse testing as well as to refuse antiretrovirals. Therefore, you should offer HIV testing universally to all pregnant women—but there is no mandatory testing of the pregnant woman without her express consent to do so. If the woman is found to be HIV-positive you cannot mandate the use of antiretrovirals even though they are safe and effective in preventing transmission of the virus from mother to child. Although from time to time, there is aberrancy in the legal system that tries to prosecute a drug-using or alcohol-using pregnant woman, the autonomy of the mother legally outweighs the safety of the fetus.

> *For example,* an HIV-positive woman comes to labor and delivery at 40 weeks of pregnancy. She has a very low CD4 count (less than 50) and a high viral load (more than 500,000). You offer her a Caesarian section and intravenous zidovudine, which can cut the transmission rate in half even on the day of delivery. The woman is anxious, but clearly has the capacity to understand the implications of this decision on both her health and the health of her child. She is still refusing the C-section and medications. What should you do next?

Fortunately this circumstance is rare and the HIV perinatal transmission rate in the United States is well under 5 percent. However, a woman's right to choose her own forms of health care are considered superior to virtually all other treatment concerns. The wrong answer in a question like this would be to give the medications anyway, to get a court order to compel the patient to take the zidovudine, to ask the father for consent for either the zidovudine or the C-section, or to sedate the patient and perform the C-section.

The autonomy of the mother is legally superior to beneficence for the fetus. Although a 40-week fetus is a viable child, the fetus is still inside the woman's body and doesn't become a person until it is delivered. A woman has the right to refuse HIV testing in pregnancy, to refuse antiretroviral medications in pregnancy, and to refuse a C-section even if it will markedly benefit the child.

PARTNER NOTIFICATION

The high level of confidentiality concerning HIV can only be breached under very specific circumstances such as when the health of a third party is at risk. A circumstance such as this would be when an HIV-positive person has a sexual or needle-sharing partner that is at risk. The method of notification follows the steps of first counseling a patient to notify his partners voluntarily. This would be ideal and follows the general theme of USMLE, which is to first answer "encourage discussions" when listed as one of the choices. If the patient is either emotionally unable or unwilling to notify their partners the next step is to notify the Department of Health to start the process of contact tracing. The health department interviews the patient and attempts to construct a list of partners in order to notify them.

This is a voluntary process and there is neither a penalty nor criminal threat of prosecution if the patient chooses not to comply. The health department then sends notice to the partner that there is a health-related issue to discuss and the partner is notified in person of their potential exposure to HIV. At this point voluntary confidential testing is offered. The name of the source patient is never revealed to the partner and the confidentiality of the original partner is maintained.

If the patient is still unwilling to disclose the names of his contacts you cannot compel him to do so. There is no incarceration or criminal penalty for not disclosing these names. If a patient will not notify his partners and you have certain knowledge of the partner at risk, you have legal immunity to carry out the notification yourself. There is legal protection if you do notify the partner, but it is not mandatory for you to do so. No one has ever been successfully prosecuted for violating a patient's confidentiality if it is to warn another person who is at risk.

> *For example,* you have a patient in your clinic who is accompanied by her boyfriend. She is clearly having unprotected sex because she is pregnant. When you ask if her boyfriend knows her HIV status she says, "Of course not—he might leave me if I told him." You have a protracted discussion about the critical importance of not putting her partner at risk. You strongly encourage her to tell him her HIV status. On a subsequent visit, when you ask her if she has notified her partner she says, "Not yet." You know the boyfriend because he accompanies her to the office visits. What should you do?

You have both a duty to the patient in terms of her health care and her confidentiality. However, you also have a duty to protect the partner. You have legal immunity if you notify the partner. At this point either you can ask the health department to notify the partner or you may do it yourself. If the partner were to seroconvert for HIV and you did not make sure he was notified you would be legally liable because you did not follow your duty to warn. This is similar to having a psychiatric patient who told you he was going to harm someone. Although you have a duty to maintain the confidentiality of the patient, you also have a duty to inform the person at risk.

HIV-POSITIVE HEALTH-CARE WORKERS

There is no duty on the part of an HIV-positive health-care worker to inform his patients of his HIV status. Universal precautions are supposed to be maintained. These should protect the patients. An HIV-positive physician who practices high-risk surgical and obstetric procedures is expected to maintain precautions to protect the patients from transmission.

REFUSAL TO TREAT HIV-POSITIVE PATIENTS

It is ethically unacceptable to refuse to treat HIV or take care of HIV-positive patients simply because they are HIV-positive. If you have a physician to whom you refer patients for various treatments, it would not be ethical for that person to discriminate only on the basis of the patient being HIV-positive. On the other hand, you cannot compel a physician to take over the management of any patient if the physician doesn't want to do so. If your question brings up the subject of refusal, the best answer is to refer the patient to someone else who will perform the care.

Chapter 10: **Sexually Transmitted Diseases (STDs)**

The ethical issues surrounding STDs have to do with partner notification, contact tracing, and reporting requirements. Although reporting requirements vary somewhat from state to state, certain diseases are reportable nationally such as syphilis, gonorrhea, and AIDS. Herpes simplex is generally not reportable and there is no contact tracing for herpes. Contact tracing is predominantly used to interrupt a cycle of transmission. Herpes cannot be eradicated from the body; hence there is no utility in treating the partner. Gonorrhea and syphilis, however, can be asymptomatically carried by the contacts of our patients and they can be transmitted to additional partners even if the source patient is asymptomatic. In addition, syphilis and gonorrhea can be eradicated (cured) with treatment.

> *For example,* 'Bob' is a 32-year-old man in your clinic being treated for primary syphilis. He is very embarrassed about his diagnosis and he asks you if his condition will be kept confidential. What should you tell him?

Just because you must contact and treat partners of patients with STDs such as syphilis does not mean you will breach his confidentiality and identify him as the source to his contacts. There is a clear order of tracing and treating his sexual contacts. If there is a choice that says "encourage him to notify his partners" or "ask if he has already told his contacts" that should be the first thing to do. If that is not a choice, then you should offer to inform the contacts for the patient if he does not want to do it. At all points you should be clear that you will not contact his partners and say, "Bob gave you a disease."

> *For example,* Bob tells you that he is not comfortable informing his partners himself and he does not want you to do it either. What should you tell him?

The Department of Health can compile a list of contacts of patients with STDs and notify the contacts that they are at risk. The Department of Health does not divulge Bob's name to the contact. The Department of Health contacts the partners and says there is an important health issue concerning them that has come to the department's attention and then asks them to come to the health department. When they arrive, the partners are told for which disease they are at risk, but they are not told the identity of the source. They are then encouraged to seek testing and treatment. The majority of patients wish to be informed, tested, and treated in order to protect their own health.

> *For example,* Bob does not want to tell either you or the Department of Health the names of his partners. He says he is monogamous now and, in fact, he is accompanied by his pregnant wife. He has not told his wife of his condition. What should you do now?

As always, you should answer "encourage him to disclose," "offer counseling for partner notification," or some statement that is gentle in terms of respecting the patient's autonomy. If these are not in the choices or the patient refuses then you must directly notify his pregnant wife immediately. Her testing and treatment is essential to protect both her own health as well as to prevent perinatal transmission. Congenital syphilis is a serious and dangerous disease but is entirely preventable.

> *For example,* you politely inform Bob that you have a duty to protect both his wife as well as his child and you are forced to notify her or have the Department of Health notify her of her risk of syphilis if he will not do it. Bob becomes furious and threatens to sue you if you violate his confidentiality. What should you tell him?

You are legally protected if you inform a person at risk of harm. In addition, there is a duty to warn people at risk of harm. Bob can get as upset as he wants. You are not legally at risk.

Chapter 11: Malpractice

DEFINITION

Malpractice is a preventable error in care of the patient resulting in harm to the patient. Malpractice is also dependent on determining if the patient's care deviated from the standard of care in a local community. In other words, if the physician did or did not do something that was different from what is locally accepted practice that resulted in harm to the patient then malpractice occurred. The intent or level of goodwill of the practitioner is not relevant if harm occurred. If a very sweet and sincere person gave fosphenytoin for congestive failure instead of furosemide because of his terrible handwriting then malpractice has occurred if the patient's condition worsened and he was harmed. If the best surgeon in the world amputates the wrong foot, then malpractice has occurred. How nice someone is has an enormous correlation with how angry patients may be, and how likely they are to file suit, but it doesn't establish liability.

> *For example,* a surgeon is consulted to place a central line. He is very rude and arrogant and speaks harshly to the patient. The patient signs consent after being informed of the complications and alternatives in management. A pneumothorax occurs and the patient is infuriated that this "high-handed bastard" hurt him. He files suit against the surgeon for malpractice. What will be the most likely outcome of the suit?

In the same way that being pleasant does not absolve you of liability, being harsh and unpleasant do not equal malpractice. A pneumothorax is an occasional complication of central line placement. The patient was fully informed of this and still agreed to the procedure. There has not automatically been wrongdoing in this case.

Evidence of harm is an important part of establishing malpractice. There must be both an error in the care, as well as evidence that there has been an adverse effect on the patient.

> *For example,* a patient with diabetes has osteomyelitis on an X ray of his foot. The physician does not perform a bone biopsy and gives the patient oral cefadroxyl for six weeks. After therapy is over, the osteomyelitis has completely resolved. The patient sees some literature on the Internet several months later conclusively showing that a bone biopsy is an indispensable part of osteomyelitis care to determine an organism and its sensitivities. In addition, he sees that intravenous therapy is the standard of care. He files suit against the physician. What will be the most likely outcome?

The patient is right that the physician deviated from the standard of care on these two points. However, his disease was effectively treated and there was no harm done to the patient, and in fact there was benefit. Therefore, malpractice has not occurred.

DEVIATIONS FROM LOCAL STANDARDS OF CARE

Physicians must practice according to accepted therapy based on demonstrated efficacy. Because there is a certain amount of subjectivity in care, it is incumbent upon the physician to determine what the locally accepted standard of care is. In addition, you must fully inform the patient of all options in care in order to make a truly informed choice.

> *For example,* a surgeon has just moved into private practice in Beverly Hills, California, after his research fellowship. His patient with lymphoma signs consent for an exploratory laparotomy to stage lymphoma. He does not inform the patient that CT scanning is a valid option. The surgeon tells her, "I don't trust those scans. We always did laparotomies in my fellowship." The patient develops an abdominal wound infection leaving her with a scar that ends her career as a swimsuit model. In the suit that follows the surgeon states, "I did the most accurate procedure for my patient to exclude cancer in the abdomen. That is what all my professors did in their studies." What will most likely be the outcome?

The surgeon erred in two ways. First, he did not explain to the patient that a CT scan of the abdomen is a valid option to exclude stage III lymphoma. Because he did not fully inform her, he will probably lose the case. Second, the local standard of care outside of certain research protocols is to do only the scans. Because the patient developed a complication from an avoidable procedure and there has been harm, the physician is at fault and will probably lose the case. The same reasoning would be true for a surgeon insisting on an axillary lymph node dissection for every patient with breast cancer instead of a sentinel lymph node dissection. If the patient develops edema and cellulitis from an unnecessary procedure, then there has been harm. The sentinel node dissection is most often the local standard of care. In addition, if the patient was not informed of the option of an axillary dissection, then there has not been full informed consent. The patient cannot choose a procedure if she has never heard of it.

INFORMED CONSENT PROTECTION AGAINST LIABILITY

Errors and complications do not automatically imply malpractice. In terms of errors, part of the liability depends on whether or not the error resulted in harm to the patient.

> *For example,* a patient admits to the hospital for a knee replacement. The staff forgets to start the patient on deep venous thrombosis (DVT) prophylaxis. The patient does not develop a DVT. On transferring care several months later the patient obtains a copy of the chart and sees the omission. He files suit for a deviation of care. What is the most likely outcome?

Although it is a clear error to omit DVT prophylaxis in this case, no harm has occurred to the patient and it would be difficult to obtain monetary reimbursement for damages if the patient is unharmed.

Complications of therapy do not imply malpractice. The main issue in determining malpractice is whether the patient was fully informed that the harm could occur and whether or not he was informed of other valid options in therapy. If he was fully informed and he signed consent anyway, then malpractice has not necessarily occurred.

> *For example,* an actress develops stage IV non-Hodgkin's lymphoma. You inform her that neither surgery nor local radiation will be appropriate. She agrees to undergo combination chemotherapy and has been informed of all the potential adverse effects including hair loss, sterility, and peripheral neuropathy. The usual and customary dose of the chemotherapy is given and the patient loses her hair and develops neuropathy from the vincristine. She is not able to work because of her appearance. She files suit because of this. What will be the most likely outcome?

Although in this case harm has occurred to the patient, the physician is not held liable for malpractice. He has fully informed the patient that her best option for survival was chemotherapy and that hair loss and neuropathy could occur. Although it is unfortunate that this has occurred, that does not make it malpractice.

INFORMED REFUSAL IS AS IMPORTANT AS INFORMED CONSENT

If a patient refuses therapy it is not sufficient to say that the patient was a competent adult who had the ability to refuse therapy. The patient must be fully informed of the effects and possible outcomes of refusing therapy including all the harm that could occur. If the patient still refuses then there has been no malpractice. It is also not acceptable to say that a patient was difficult, abusive, or unable to understand English. The physician has an obligation to provide information to adult patients with decision-making capacity in a language that they can understand.

> *For example,* a 60-year-old man comes to the emergency department with one hour of chest pain and an ST segment elevation myocardial infarction. The patient is a recent immigrant who speaks French and understands little English. You inform the patient that the best therapy is angioplasty and possibly thrombolytics. You explain that they can develop intracranial bleeding from the thrombolytics and a hematoma at the site of the catheter placement from the angioplasty. The patient, anxious to avoid these complications, refuses both. You do not double check the refusal with a translator. The patient dies and his family sues you for malpractice. In your defense you point out the clear fact that you offered the patient lifesaving therapy and he refused. What will be the most likely outcome?

In addition to informing a patient of the complications of therapy, you must also inform them of the complications of not receiving the therapy. In addition, if there is the question of a language problem, you must obtain a translator to double check your patient understands the impact of withholding the treatment. In this case it was not documented that you told the patient that he could die without the treatment. He was not fully informed. You would lose the lawsuit.

PATIENTS MUST FULLY INFORM THE PHYSICIAN OF THEIR MEDICAL PROBLEMS

For example, a man is admitted for a possible DVT. He denies any past medical history. He does not inform you of his recent diagnosis of a gastric ulcer after endoscopy for severe upper gastrointestinal bleeding. There is no previous record at this hospital. You give him heparin and he hemorrhages massively. He sues you for harming him. His lawyer knows you gave heparin to a patient with a history of bleeding that harmed the patient. What will be the most likely outcome?

In addition to a patient's right to be fully informed of the risks and benefits of therapy, the patient also has a responsibility to inform you of their entire medical history. There is no malpractice if the patient has a complication from a previous illness that he did not tell you about and you had no way of knowing of. If the patient has a history of an allergy to penicillin and he does not tell you when you ask, you are not held liable if you administer penicillin and he develops an allergic reaction.

RISK MANAGEMENT

Risk management is the term applied to the administrative portion of the hospital devoted to assessing liability issues in terms of care. Risk management assesses deviations in care and analyzes cases in which wrongdoing might have occurred in order to minimize the risk of litigation for the hospital.

MEDICAL ERRORS

The physician has a duty to inform patients of errors in care if those errors will have an impact on the patient's care. The patient has a right to know what is happening in his management. This includes all errors that may affect the outcome of the patient's care. Informing the patient is not limited just to telling him about the errors that you know he will find out about or to inform him just about the ones that may result in litigation and malpractice. If I bring my car to you for repair and your assistant breaks the windshield by mistake, I have a right to be informed. The car is my property and I have a right to know what is happening with it.

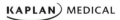

On the other hand there is no mandate to inform a patient about minor errors that will have no impact on her care or treatment. If the blood tests were delayed or a single test forgotten the patient does not have to be informed of this as long as the information is obtained in a timely fashion and as long as it will not impact her care. The main determinant of the need to inform the patient is not the magnitude of the mistake, but rather the impact on her life and health care.

Chapter 12: **Doctor/Patient Relationship**

BEGINNING AND ENDING THE RELATIONSHIP

The relationship between a doctor and his patient is a voluntary relationship that is to be entered freely on both sides. In the same way that you cannot compel a patient to accept a particular doctor as her physician without her agreement, a physician cannot be compelled to accept a patient without his agreement. A doctor must agree to accept a patient. There is no obligation on the part of the physician to accept a patient. This is true no matter what need the patient has and whatever expertise the doctor may possess.

> *For example,* a patient with diabetes lives in a small town with only one endocrinologist. The endocrinologist has a full practice and is not accepting new patients. The patient has very bad diabetes and has a very complex regimen that her family practitioner insists is beyond the scope of his understanding. The patient shows up in the office and insists to the office manager that she be accepted. What should be done?

The physician is under no legal obligation to accept the patient. There is considerable misunderstanding of this issue. The physician, by training and inclination, is geared to aid the suffering. However, there is still no mandate for the physician to accept the patient nor can a patient force a physician to take care of her. Even Good Samaritan laws, which protects caregivers from liability if they aid a sick person in the street, do not force the doctor to aid an injured person. You may feel a moral obligation to help everyone, but there is no legal obligation to enter into a doctor/patient relationship. This is different from a hospital's mandate to provide emergency treatment to anyone who comes to the emergency department. Hospitals cannot turn anyone away at the door of their emergency room if they come seeking care. This does not mean they must provide continuous care after discharge, but it does mean there is a national legal mandate for all hospitals to provide emergency management and treatment of all patients.

Once a patient and physician have entered into a care relationship there is far greater complexity in ending that relationship. A physician cannot suddenly end the relationship. He must maintain the care of the patient until the patient can find an appropriate alternate source of care and he must give "reasonable notice".

GIFTS FROM PATIENTS

Small gifts from patients of nominal or modest value are acceptable on the part of the physician. This is provided that there is no expectation of a different form of therapy or a higher level of care based on the gift. You can accept a cake at Christmas, a balloon on your birthday, or other tokens of esteem, but not if the patient expects an extra, or different prescription for something, in exchange for the gift.

The rules on gifts from patients are far less rigorous, precise, or clear than the rules on gifts from the pharmaceutical industry. There is an automatic presumption that gifts from industry always carry an influence toward a product, service, or prescribing practice. Gifts from industry are viewed differently because there can be no other intention behind them except to buy influence and alter behavior. There is no such automatic presumption on the part of gifts received from patients.

DOCTOR/PATIENT SEXUAL CONTACT

Sexual contact between a physician and a patient is always inappropriate. It is unclear if there can ever be a completely acceptable, ethical way to alter the physician/patient relationship so that sexual contact is acceptable. At the very least, the physician and patient must mutually agree to end the formal professional relationship of a doctor and a patient. It is not clear how much time must elapse between the ending of the professional doctor/patient relationship and the beginning of a personal relationship. The recommendation for psychiatrists is somewhat unique. The American Psychiatric Association guidelines specifically state that there can never be a sexual or personally intimate private relationship between doctor and patient even after the professional relationship has ended. In other words, a psychiatrist should not have sexual contact even with former patients.

These guidelines apply no matter who initiates the relationship. In other words, it is not more acceptable for a doctor and patient to have sexual relations if the patient initiates the sexual relationship rather than the physician. These guidelines also take no account of gender or sexual orientation. It is always ethically unacceptable to have a sexual relationship between a psychiatrist and either a current or a former patient. It is ethically unacceptable for a physician of any kind to have a sexual relationship with a current patient.

Chapter 13: **Doctor and Society**

CHILD ABUSE

Physicians are mandatory reporters of child abuse. This means that the physician has a duty to report child abuse even if they feel uncomfortable doing so. There is no discretion on whether or not to report abuse. In addition, even suspected child abuse must be reported. The reporting to child protective services should happen immediately so that there can be an urgent intervention to prevent further abuse.

> *For example,* a 20-year-old woman brings her seven-year-old son into the emergency department for a broken arm. The child has been to the emergency department twice before for various injuries. The mother lives with her boyfriend who is not the child's father. You have no direct proof that abuse has occurred and the mother simply states that the child is accident prone. When you ask her whether her domestic partner may be injuring the child she becomes very angry and vigorously denies it. What should you do?

Report suspected child abuse cases no matter what the family says. The child abuse laws are very specific in terms of protecting the mandatory reporter against liability. Even if there is no abuse found, the suspected abuser has no standing to file suit against you as long as you make the report in good faith. In other words, as long as you are sincerely and honestly making the report there is no liability on your end. Although physicians are mandatory reporters, anyone who has a good reason to suspect child abuse can make a report as long as the same criteria are operating. You must have a reason to suspect the abuse and there must be no element of trying to harm or embarrass the family.

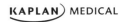

ELDER ABUSE

The same criteria described for child abuse generally apply to elder abuse. Instead of child protective services, there are adult protective services. Reports made in good faith can be done without liability to the reporter. The circumstances with elder abuse are less clear than with child abuse, because the elderly person is often a still-competent adult who may object to the report of the abuse on the basis that they are afraid of repercussions in the home or the loss of the home. Nevertheless, you must report elder abuse, and partially breaching the confidentiality of the patient and family is permissible in the interest of protecting a vulnerable person.

The other reason that elder abuse reporting is less clear is that there is no uniform national standard for it in all 50 states. The vast majority of states, however, have a reporting system similar to that for reporting child abuse. The bottom line for USMLE is that you should answer to "report the abuse to adult protective services" if the case is presented.

IMPAIRED DRIVERS

The rules on reporting impaired drivers vary enormously nationally. There is no other aspect of medical ethics and health-care legality that has such state-to-state variability as the management of the impaired driver. All states require the patient to report seizure disorders; however the period of time that the driver must stay off the road varies vastly from one state to another and therefore cannot be tested on the USMLE.

Physicians cannot suspend driving privileges. Only the state-sponsored Department of Motor Vehicles (DMV) can suspend or revoke driving privileges. When a driver is impaired in any way, the first step is to encourage the driver to report the impairment, to the DMV. In addition, the physician should encourage all impaired drivers to limit or curtail their driving. There is no uniform agreement of what, beside seizure disorders and visual impairment should be reported in all states. Only a few states have specific laws requiring reporting of syncopal episodes. Not all states offer immunity to physicians, such as the protections offered for reporting child abuse, for reporting an impaired driver.

> *For example,* you are the attending physician on a patient admitted to the hospital with a first-time seizure. The head CT and EEG are normal. You will not be starting antiseizure medications. The patient drives to work regularly. What should you do concerning the patient's ability to drive?

Mandatory self-reporting of seizures is required in all 50 states. If there is an answer that says "encourage refraining from driving" or "counsel on alternate forms of transportation," that is the best thing to do first. If that is not one of the answers then choose "recommend the patient inform the DMV" is the best choice.

> *For example,* you are evaluating an 87-year-old man in your office for markedly worsening cognitive dysfunction. He is on a number of cardiac medications as well that leave him somewhat dizzy. There is evidence of psychomotor retardation and delayed reaction time on your examination. You are concerned that the patient regularly drives. What should you do about his driving?

If the patient does not have a specific disease such as a seizure disorder that makes him potentially unsafe, then it is much less clear what your responsibilities are toward both the patient as well as to society. In cases like this the best answer is to recommend that the patient with cognitive problems curtail his driving or find alternate forms of transportation. Given that the reporting requirements are so variable on a state-to-state basis this is often the best answer that would be uniformly true in all states.

> *For example,* you have a 65-year-old man with progressive glaucoma in your office. His vision is severely impaired and getting worse. You strongly doubt that he can read traffic signs on the highway. You have repeatedly encouraged him to curtail his driving but he has not. What is your responsibility toward this patient?

In those cases where the patient's visual acuity is so severely impaired that you suspect he is a danger to himself and to others when driving, you must strongly encourage the patient to stop driving. You can intervene directly in the states that require intact vision for recertification of the driver's license by refusing to provide recertification. In those cases where this is not possible you must inform the patient that it is your duty to notify the DMV of his impairment. You do not have the right to remove or suspend driving privileges. You do, however, have a duty to report a visually impaired driver to the DMV so that the DMV may make its own determination of whether the patient's license should be removed or limited.

PHYSICIAN PARTICIPATION IN EXECUTIONS

A physician cannot ethically participate in executions in prisons. This is true even though the execution is legal in that state. Participating as a physician in any way in an execution directly opposes the eithical imperative to preserve life. The physician's ethical duty to relieve suffering and to protect life supersedes any ability to participate in the execution.

> ***For example,*** you are a physician in a state prison. The warden has asked your assistance in checking the apparatus that delivers a lethal injection scheduled for use in an execution tomorrow. He is not asking you to administer the injection. You have never met the patient before and you have no prior doctor/patient relationship with the condemned prisoner. What should you tell the warden?

A physician cannot participate in any way in an execution as a physician. Participating in an execution impairs your physician/patient relationships with the other prisoners who are your patients. It is ethically impermissible to participate even at the level of a technical consultant—even if you have no doctor/patient relationship with the prisoner. You may not give the injection, start the IV line, mix the medications for injection, or design the formulation for the lethal injection. It is not even permissible for you to certify that death has occurred unless another party has determined it first.

TORTURE

Physicians cannot participate in torture at any level. The knowledge of torture must be reported and opposed as you would report and oppose elder abuse, child abuse, or an impaired driver. You may treat those injured by torture once the victims have been removed from an environment where torture may occur; you cannot treat injuries to allow patients to become well enough to withstand more torture.

USMLE is likely to expand its coverage of questions on the military physician. The bottom line is that medical ethics for a physician are considered to take precedence over any form of employment even if it is in the military. This means that participation in torture at any level is always considered unethical. Torture or 'harsh interrogation practices' are to be considered the equivalent of child abuse. You are required to report any such events you know of. This also includes being a physician in a legal war zone or while under the direct orders of a military superior. In all of these cases, your ethical duty a physician takes precedence over the superior in any other organizational structure.

SPOUSAL ABUSE

The ethics and legalities surrounding spousal abuse are somewhat different from those for child abuse and elder abuse. In the case of spousal abuse, you are dealing with an adult patient that is generally competent consequently you do not have the same authority to report the abuse against the wishes of the victim as you would in a case of child abuse. Many victims experiencing spousal abuse believe they are not in a position to be able to leave the relationship or to report the abuse for fear of worse abuse. Consequently you cannot report the abuse to the police or to anyone else without the express consent of the victim.

> *For example,* a 45-year-old woman comes to the emergency department after having had her nose broken by her husband. She has been abused several times in the past. When you tell her you will report the injury to the police she becomes very anxious and insists you tell no one because her husband is a police officer. What should you do?

When the patient will not give consent to have the injury reported, you should answer that you will "encourage the victim to report" or "offer counseling."

GUNSHOT WOUNDS

Reporting of gunshot wounds is mandatory but from a different perspective than the other forms of reporting. The mandatory reporting of gunshot wounds is based on pursuing a criminal investigation of the person doing the shooting. Report a gunshot wound even if the victim objects. The societal need for safety supersedes the privacy of the patient in the case of gunshots.

GIFTS AND INDUSTRY FUNDING

Gifts from industry are to be limited in both type and by numerical monetary value. The presumption is that all gifts from industry are an indirect attempt to obtain influence from physicians in terms of their prescribing patterns. Modest gifts of less than $100 in value are acceptable only if they are medical or educational in nature. In other words, you can receive $100 worth of books or medical equipment but you cannot just get a $100 check for cash. In addition, the industry may sponsor educational presentations as long as they do not interfere with the content. Physicians may accept meals that are in association with educational experiences such as lectures or conferences.

Physicians are prohibited from accepting gifts from the industry that are purely geared to enhance the income of the physician or merely for entertainment. For example, the physician cannot accept tickets to basketball games or other sporting events, theater tickets, ski trips, or gift certificates to department stores.

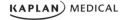

Chapter 14: **Doctor/Doctor Relationship**

REPORTING IMPAIRED PHYSICIANS

Physicians have as much of a duty to report an impaired physician as they do to report child abuse. Although enormously confrontational, there is no discretion in terms of avoiding reporting an impaired physician when the impairment is clear. If you know that another physician is not functioning normally and may be a danger to patients, the privacy of the physician is less important than the safety of his patients. This is true whether the impairment is from substance abuse, a psychiatric disorder, Alzheimer's disease, or an emotional disturbance.

You should report physicians and students-in-training to their local supervisor first; report a resident to his program director or department chair; and report a medical student to his dean or course director. You should report attending physicians to the department chair or division head. If the attending physician is a self-employed physician in private practice, then there is no department chair or division head to which you can make a report. You should report physicians in the community in private practice to the state board of medical conduct or the state health or education department. The key is to go to whoever might have authority over that physician. The lines of supervision are much clearer in the hospital or in medical school, where there are clear supervisors.

> *For example,* Dr. Smith is an attending in endocrinology that is doing a month as the attending on the general medical service at King's County Hospital in Brooklyn. Unfortunately, his house staff finds him getting lost on the way to the bathroom in the hospital. In addition, he has no knowledge of general medical practice and he can't remember the cases after the residents present them. The senior resident on service mentions this to you and asks your advice about what to do given that Alzheimer's might be developing. What should you tell him?

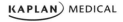

The resident has a duty to report the potentially impaired physician to the department chair. This will allow for a private, confidential intervention with the attending physician. It can allow for an evaluation that can determine if the physician is truly impaired. It is possible that an impaired physician could have a correctable problem that might not otherwise come to light without this report. In addition, the rates of substance abuse for physicians are the same as the rates of substance abuse for the general population. Reporting the impaired physician may be the only way of getting a doctor into treatment for his substance abuse. Catching substance abuse before patient harm occurs prevents malpractice. The physician can be successfully rehabilitated and returned to practice.

You only have a duty to report behavior that affects patient care. If a physician goes out to wild parties but there is no detectable impairment of patient care, this is not something to report. If a physician likes to get tattoos, use bad language, and ride in a motorcycle gang on the weekend, this is not something to report. Your duty to report is based exclusively on behaviors found to have an adverse effect on patient care.

The bottom line is that it is your mandatory duty to report an impaired physician who may potentially be a danger to patients. You have the same protections for yourself on reporting as you do in child abuse, which is that there is no penalty if the report is found to be untrue as long as the report is made in good faith without malice.

PHYSICIAN DISAGREEMENTS

If an attending physician disagrees with a resident's improper management, there is little problem because the attending physician has the authority to overrule the resident. It is much more problematic if the resident disagrees with the attending physician.

If the resident finds what may be an error in management with the attending physician, the USMLE first wants you to answer "discuss," "confer," or "try to reach consensus with evidence-based medicine." If these discussions are not satisfactory, then bring the issue to whatever is the version of a higher authority locally. The key words are "higher" and "locally." Do not go straight to the state medical board, licensing board, or governing body without first trying to have a discussion with the division head or department chair. In addition, do not answer "Inform the patient."

What if the resident is wrong? Disagreements between physicians are handled in much the same way as the reporting an impaired physician is handled, except that you should always first pursue discussion with the person with whom you are disagreeing. You cannot make changes in a patient's care without the attending physician knowing and approving the changes. The attending physician ultimately has all the responsibility for the patients, and has an absolute right to direct the care of the patients and know what is going on.

Chapter 15: **Experimentation**

RESEARCH AND EXPERIMENTATION-PARTICIPATION CONSENT

In most ways, the consent issues for participation in experimentation and research are not very different from those surrounding any other medical treatment or procedure. The research subject must be fully informed of the potential risks of the intervention as well as the possible benefits. The subject or participant must be entering the trial voluntarily—without coercion. If the subject is not an adult or lacks the capacity to understand the risk of the trial, then a valid surrogate such as a parent or guardian must give consent.

The difference between participating in experimentation and receiving a treatment is that the study medication may be given in a way that is known, in advance, to have no benefit and the subject is participating simply out of other motives to advance the accumulation of scientific data. The bottom line on experimentation is that participation must be voluntary.

PRISONER PARTICIPATION

The same rules apply to the participation of prisoners in research as apply to nonprisoners. Prisoners have the same right of refusal and informed consent. There is to be no removal or abridgement of rights simply because the patient is a prisoner.

INSTITUTIONAL REVIEW BOARD (IRB)

An Institutional Review Board (IRB) is an independent reviewing body that evaluates investigational protocols prior to their implementation to ensure their validity and ethical integrity. The IRB is comprised of representatives of different areas of the hospital or medical school that include clinicians, educators, ethicists, clergy, and scientists.

The idea is to have a broad-based group that can evaluate not only the scientific parameters of a protocol, but also ensure that the process of informed consent is accurate and that the treatments and procedures being studied do not present an undue risk to the patients being enrolled. The IRB also ensures periodic review of the data so that a trial can be stopped early on occasion. A study cannot commence within an institution without IRB approval.

> *For example,* a group of investigators studying the effects of antiretroviral medications on patients with HIV/AIDS submits their study to the IRB for review and approval prior to implementation. The planned protocol is to study whether giving antiretroviral medications to patients with AIDS makes a difference in their outcome when compared to starting the medications after discharge.

Half the patients will receive a placebo and the other half will receive the antiretroviral medications. The study will randomize patients admitted to the hospital for acute opportunistic infections. The IRB rejects the study on the basis that it would not be ethical to withhold potentially lifesaving therapy from a group of patients in which the efficacy has already been proven. In addition, the IRB rejects the study because the consent form was not translated into Spanish.

The IRB's purpose is also to make sure that a study seeks to answer valid questions. It is not valid to withhold proven effective therapy to gather data on how some patients are harmed just to produce a publication. There is no randomized, placebo-controlled trial proving that antibiotics are better than placebo in patients with severe pneumonia. This is because the concept of the randomized trial has only been in existence since the second half of the 20th century. Because Penicillin was already the standard of care for pneumonia, it would have been unethical to perform a study in which antibiotics were withheld from patients with pneumonia and to watch these patients die. It would also be unethical to do a study of steroids in minimal change nephrotic syndrome when the efficacy is clear.

The IRB is a response to the Nuremberg War Crimes Tribunal, during which the world consensus that experimentation without consent is unethical and not allowable became clear. Nazi experimentation during World War II was coerced, without consent of the participants, and collected data that involved the unnecessary and willful harm of human subjects. The modern IRB is the method of ensuring safety, ethical integrity, and freedom from coercion in clinical investigation.

FINANCIAL DISCLOSURE

When investigators publish or present research data, disclosure of all relevant sources of financing for the work is required. If I am publishing a study comparing two different anti-retroviral medications, it is important to disclose to the audience in a Grand Rounds that I have received funding from antiretroviral manufacturers. If I am publishing a study on an implantable defibrillator, it is mandatory that I reveal that I own part of the company that manufactures the equipment. Financial disclosure is essential to help ensure an objective interpretation of research data.

The reason for double-blind placebo controlled trials is that we know that the desire of the people running the study and collecting the data can influence the study results.

Disclosure of financing helps understand a possible bias in a study. The most important modern example is an article in the journal *The Lancet* on the dangers of the measles vaccination. In addition to many other flaws in the study, the author failed to disclose, and *The Lancet* failed to investigate, the financial arrangement of the author with a rival vaccine manufacturer. The study was invalid, although published, because the author was attempting to invalidate a current measles vaccine in hopes of acquiring approval for the marketing and reimbursement of his own vaccine. This is an excellent example of why financial disclosure can help preserve scientific integrity.

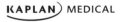

Practice Questions

BRAIN DEATH

1. An 80-year-old man is admitted to the hospital with a massive intracranial bleed. He has been placed on a ventilator because of the respiratory failure associated with intracranial herniation. When you try to remove the ventilator, there are no respirations. The patient makes no purposeful movements. There is no pupilary reaction when you shine a light in his eyes. There is no nystagmus on cold caloric testing. Oculocephalic and corneal reflexes are absent. He left no specific wishes for his care.

   Which of the following is the most appropriate action regarding this patent?

    a. Remove the ventilator.

   b. Make the patient DNR.

   c. Place a nasogastric tube to prevent aspiration.

   d. Get a court order authorizing you to remove the ventilator.

   e. Do an EEG (electroencephalogram) three times separated by six hours each time.

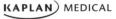

CHILD ABUSE

2. You are a resident in the emergency department. An irate parent comes to you furious because the social worker has been asking him about striking his child. The child is a 5-year-old boy who has been in the emergency department four times this year with several episodes of trauma that did not seem related. Today, the child is brought in with a child complaint of "slipping into a hot bathtub" with a burn wound on his legs. The parent threatens to sue you and says "How dare you think that about me? I love my son!"

    What should you do?

    a. Give reassurance to the parents and treat the patient's injury appropriately.

    b. Ask risk management to evaluate the case.

    c. Admit the child to remove him from the possibly dangerous environment.

    d. Call the police.

    e. Ask the father yourself if there has been any abuse.

    f. Speak to the wife privately about possible episodes of abuse.

    g. Explain to the parents that the next time this happens you will have to call child protective services.

    h. Report the family to child protective services.

    i. Give the parents a referral to a family therapist they can see with the child the following week.

CONFIDENTIALITY

3. You are working at the desk in your hospital when another employee of the hospital asks for information about a patient who was admitted last night with a pulmonary embolus secondary to cancer. You know the details of the case. The person requesting the information states that he is a close friend and co-worker of your patient. He shows you proper identification proving he really is a co-worker of your patient who also works in the hospital.

   Which of the following is the most appropriate response to this request?

   a. Give him the information on the patient.

   b. Give him the information only if he is a relative of the patient.

   c. Inform him that you are not at liberty to give details regarding the patient without the patient's permission.

   d. Have him sign a release or consent form before revealing the information.

4. You are seeing patients in clinic when two men in dark suits and dark glasses come in and show you badges marking them as members of a federal law enforcement agency. The identification is legitimate. These "men in black" inform you that they are making a "minor investigation" of one of your patients. They ask to look at the patient's chart for a few minutes, saying, "You wouldn't want to interfere with a federal investigation, would you?"

   What should you do?

   a. Give them the chart.

   b. Give them the chart but watch what they do with it.

   c. Ask them to sign a release for the chart so you are absolved of responsibility.

   d. Tell them you cannot show them the chart unless there is a signed release from the patient.

   e. Tell them that you can give copies but not the original record.

   f. Don't give them the chart but read the relevant information to them.

KAPLAN) MEDICAL

5. You are a psychiatrist in session with a patient who tells you he thinks his boss at work is persecuting him. The patient has had mild schizophrenia. The patient asks you if you can keep a secret and then tells you that he is planning to kill his boss "when the time is right." You say, "Of course, everything you tell me during the session will always be confidential."

   What should you do?

   a. Keep the patient's session confidential but make attempts to discourage the patient from his plan.

   b. Inform your medical director and let him handle it.

   c. Inform law enforcement agencies of the threat to the patient's boss.

   d. Inform the patient's boss that he is in danger.

   e. Inform both the patient's boss as well as law enforcement of the threat.

6. You are discussing the care of an elderly woman with her family. Although she is awake and alert, the patient is very ill and physically fragile. You are awaiting the results of a biopsy for what will likely be cancer, which has already metastasized throughout the body. The family asks that you inform them first about the results of the biopsy. They are very loving and caring and are constantly surrounding the patient. They do not want to depress the patient further, and because there will be no hope for a cure they see no reason to ruin her remaining life with this information.

   What should you tell them?

   a. You will honor their wishes.

   b. You agree with their wishes and you ask them to give you the necessary written request.

   c. You ask them to involve the ethics committee for the hospital.

   d. You tell them that you are obligated to inform the patient of all the findings.

   e. Explain to them that that decision can only be made by the health-care proxy.

7. Your patient has just recently been diagnosed with familial adenomatous polyposis (FAP). This disorder is chronic, progressive, and fatal. There is a genetic test that can tell whether children of parents with the disease will develop it. The test is very accurate. The patient has become divorced and refuses to give you his consent to inform his ex-wife who now has custody of their three children. He threatens to sue you if you reveal elements of his medical care to his ex-wife.

What should you do?

a. Respect the patient's right to confidentiality.

b. Transfer the patient's care to another physician as long as the patient agrees.

c. Ask the health department to inform the patient's ex-wife about the disease risk.

d. Seek a court order to inform the patient's ex-wife.

e. Inform the patient's ex-wife of the risk to the children.

f. Inform the ex-wife's doctor.

8. You are seeing a patient in clinic who has developed tuberculosis. He is an undocumented (illegal) immigrant. His family will need to be screened for tuberculosis with PPD skin testing. He is frightened of being deported if the Department of Health learns his immigration status.

What should you tell him?

a. "Don't worry, the Department of Health does not ask for or report immigration status."

b. "Only people who are noncompliant with medications are reported to the government."

c. "Don't worry, I will fully treat you before we deport you."

d. "I am sorry but there is nothing I can do about it; there is mandatory reporting to the government.

DONATION OF ORGANS

9. A couple comes to see you after having tried in-vitro fertilization and artificial insemination. They are very happy because they have recently been successful in giving birth to a child. They have a significant amount of leftover sperm, eggs, and some fertilized gametes/embryos and they are thinking about selling them.

   What should you tell them?

   a. It is legal to sell only the eggs.

   b. It is legal to sell only the sperm.

   c. It is legal to sell both the sperm and eggs but not the embryos.

   d. It is illegal to sell any of them.

   e. It is legal to sell all of them.

10. You are a fourth-year medical student with a patient who has been in a severe motor vehicle accident. The patient has a subdural hematoma that led to cerebral herniation before it could be drained. Over the last few days, the patient has lost all brainstem reflexes and is now brain dead. You have the closest relationship with the family of anyone on the team. The ventilator is to be removed soon and organ donation is considered.

    Who should ask for consent for organ donation in this case?

    a. You, because you are the person with the best relationship with the family

    b. The resident because you are only a student

    c. Attending of record

    d. Hospital administration

    e. Organ-donor network

11. A 50-year-old male gambler owes money to everyone and is seeking a rapid source of cash. He answers an advertisement in a foreign newspaper offering $30,000 for one of his kidneys. He comes to see you for medical evaluation prior to the approval to be a donor.

    What should you tell him?

    a. It is never acceptable to receive any money for solid organs or bone marrow.
    b. It is acceptable as long as the recipient truly need the organ.
    c. It is okay as long as the donor's remaining kidney is healthy.
    d. It is acceptable if the surgery for both the donation as well at the implantation in the recipient is occurring in a foreign country.
    e. Reimbursement for cost of travel and lodging for the donation is acceptable, but profiting from the donation is unacceptable.

12. A man arrives at the emergency department on a ventilator after an accident. He is brain dead by all criteria. He has an organ-donor card in his wallet indicating his desire to donate. The organ-donor team contacts the family. The family refuses to sign consent for the donation.

    What should be done?

    a. Remove the organs anyway.
    b. Wait for the patient's heart to stop and then remove the organs.
    c. Stop the ventilator and remove the organs.
    d. Seek a court order to overrule the family.
    e. Honor the wishes of the family; no donation.

DNR ORDERS

13. You have a patient with severe multiple sclerosis that is advanced and progressive who now develops renal failure secondary to diabetes. The patient is alert and has elected to put the DNR order in place at her own discretion. The patient's potassium level is now markedly elevated at 8 meq/L.

    Which of the following is the most appropriate management of this patient?

    a. Dialysis cannot be done because of the DNR order.

    b. You can do the dialysis if the DNR is reversed for the procedure.

    c. Go ahead with the dialysis; ignore the DNR order.

    d. Give kayexalate until the DNR status is discussed with the family.

14. A patient from a skilled-nursing facility is admitted to the hospital for severe upper gastrointestinal bleeding. The patient has a DNR order in place. The bleeding has not stopped despite multiple transfusions, octreotide, proton pump inhibitors, and endoscopy. He needs monitoring and evaluation in an intensive care unit.

    What should you do?

    a. Reverse the DNR order and transfer to the ICU as needed.

    b. You cannot be DNR and be in the ICU.

    c. Transfer to the ICU as needed; okay to be DNR in the ICU.

    d. He can go to the ICU with the DNR but cannot go to surgery.

    e. He can go to the ICU with the DNR but cannot be intubated.

15. A man is admitted for acute appendicitis. He is elderly and has had a home DNR order in place since he had a previous admission for another reason last year. He needs urgent surgery for the appendicitis. He still wishes to be DNR.

    What should you do about the surgery?

    a. No surgery can be done with a patient who is DNR.

    b. Reverse the DNR order for the surgery.

    c. DNR is acceptable only if the surgery does not require intubation.

    d. Surgery is acceptable while DNR if an additional consent is signed.

    e. DNR does not preclude surgery; proceed with the appendectomy.

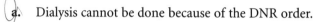

ELDER ABUSE

16. An 84-year-old woman is seen by you in clinic for routine management of her multiple medical problems. She comes alone and you notice that she has been losing weight and has several contusions. She is a widow and lives with her granddaughter and her granddaughter's husband who recently lost his job. On questioning she tells you that her granddaughter's husband does occasionally strike her when he is drunk.

What should you do?

   a. Report the abuse only at her specific request.

   b. Arrange for a meeting with your patient and the grandson-in-law.

   c. Remove the patient from the home and place her in an adult home.

   d. Have a home health aid placed to keep an eye on the patient.

   e. Arrange for an order of protection from the police.

   f. Report the grandson-in-law's abuse to adult protective service.

   g. Speak directly to the grandson-in-law about the problem.

EXECUTIONS

17. You are the staff physician in a state penitentiary in a state where capital punishment is legal. An execution is in process and the warden calls you because the technician is unable to start the intravenous line that is necessary for the lethal injection. The warden wants you to start the line and supervise the pharmacist.

What should you tell him?

   a. "No problem, I will start the line right away."

   b. "I can start the line, but I cannot push the medications."

   c. "I can start the line, but I cannot prepare or inject the medications."

   d. 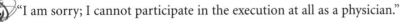"I am sorry; I cannot participate in the execution at all as a physician."

   e. "I can take care of all of it."

EXPERIMENTATION

18. You are preparing a clinical trial of different doses of a certain medication. This medication has already been proven to be clinically effective and is already approved by the Food and Drug Administration (FDA). You are only studying to see whether a higher dose of the medication will lead to enhanced benefit.

    Which of the following is true concerning your study?

    a. Institutional review board (IRB) approval is not necessary.

    b. Informed consent is required to participate.

    c. Informed consent is not required because the medication has already been FDA-approved.

    d. Informed consent is not required because you are trying to demonstrate benefit, not harm.

19. Which of the following most accurately describes the participation of prisoners in clinical trials and research?

    a. There is no need for informed consent.

    b. No monetary compensation may occur.

    c. Prisoners are not permitted to participate as research subjects.

    d. Their rights are identical to those of a nonprisoner.

    e. Research on prisoners is always considered unethical.

    f. Participation in research is an accepted means of winning early release from prison.

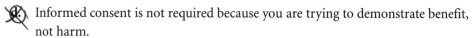

20. You are in the process of finalizing the results of your research for publication. You are the principal investigator of a clinical trial studying the effects of HMG-CoA reductase inhibitors on cardiac mortality. A prominent manufacturer of one of these medications provided major funding for the study.

    Which of the following is the most accurate in an ethical preparation for authorship of the publication?

    a. Accepting money from a company prohibits you from being listed as an author.

    b. Funding source has no impact on publication requirements.

    c. You can be listed as the author after the institutional review board checks the paper for evidence of bias.

    d. There are no restrictions on your authorship as long as you disclose the financial affiliation.

    e. There are no requirements as long as the data are accurate.

    f. You do not have to do anything as long as the checks were written to the institution and not to you.

21. Which of the following most accurately describes the primary role of an institutional review board (IRB)?

    a. Protect the institution from liability

    b. Protect the physician from liability

    c. Ensure the ethical and humane treatment of human subjects in experimentation

    d. Ensure the study is scientifically accurate

    e. Ensure that the study is financially feasible for the institution

KAPLAN MEDICAL

GENETIC TESTING

22. A 35-year-old female patient comes to your office with a large form to be filled out certifying that her health is within normal limits. This is as a part of pre-employment evaluation and is required in order for the patient to get the job. The form also asks for the results of the patient's APC (adenomatous polyposis coli) gene. This is in order for the company to determine which of its long-term employees will need expensive care. What should be your response?

    a. Perform the test.

    b. Perform the test, but do not share the results with the employer.

    c. Do not perform the test.

    d. Ask the patient if she wants the test performed and the results reported.

    e. Perform the colonoscopy; the employer is entitled to know about current health problems but not future ones.

    f. Include the test only if the patient has family members with colon cancer.

23. You have a patient with a strong family history of breast cancer. As a matter of the patient's request, you perform a BRCA genetic test to see if there is an increased risk for breast cancer. The patient's employer is requesting a copy of any genetic testing that may have been done.

    What should you do?

    a. Give the employer the information.

    b. Refer the employer to the hospital lawyer.

    c. Bring the request to the ethics committee.

    d. Refuse to provide the information to the employer.

    e. Give the information if it is positive on a repeat exam.

GIFTS

24. You are a resident invited to a dinner given by a pharmaceutical company. In addition to the dinner there is a lecture given on a medical subject as well as a $500 gift certificate to a department store for attending the presentation.

    Which of the following is the most appropriate action in this case?

    a. It is entirely unethical to accept any of it; refuse everything.

    b. It is only ethical to attend the lecture.

    c. Do not accept the money, but the dinner and the lecture are ethically acceptable.

    d. You may accept all three components.

    e. Cash payments from industry are acceptable as long as they are not tied to prescribing specific medications.

    f. You can accept because you are a resident and not an attending.

25. You have been asked to give Grand Rounds at a hospital. A manufacturer of a new medical device is sponsoring you. In exchange, you are being offered a $1,000 fee for your talk.

    What should you do?

    a. You must refuse the money.

    b. You may accept only as long as you donate it to charity.

    c. You may accept as long as you don't reveal the honorarium to the audience.

    d. It is permissible to take the money as long as you disclose any other financial or business connection with this or any other company.

    e. You may accept the money as long as you submit the content of your talk to an independent panel for review to ensure objectivity.

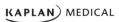

26. You have been taking care of a patient admitted with palpitations from a panic attack. He is somewhat hypomanic with pressured speech, anxiety, and flight of ideas. After several days he is feeling much better and he is extremely grateful for your help. He is quite wealthy and he offers to borrow five million dollars from the bank "to help you with your research."

    What should you tell him?

    a. "I accept!"

    b. "Thank you very much, but I cannot accept."

    c. "I accept, but only for a study of bipolar disorder."

    d. "I would be happy to take your money, but I must have you evaluated by psychiatry first."

27. You have a patient in your clinic who is an elderly woman with multiple medical problems. Her family is extremely grateful for your care and they bring you a meal they cooked at home, a cake, and a scarf.

    What should you do?

    a. Accept the gift but report it.

    b. Accept the gift.

    c. Offer payment for the food.

    d. Refuse the gift.

    e. It is ethical to accept the gift if you share the food with the rest of the house staff.

    f. Accept the food but not the scarf.

28. You have been invited to participate in a "Medical Jeopardy" game sponsored by a pharmaceutical manufacturer. The winners are to receive $100 gift certificates to the medical school's bookstore. All of the participants are to receive a stethoscope. The audience and all the participants are offered a free meal.

    Which of the following is most appropriate to accept?

    a. All the gifts

    b. Only the meal

    c. Only the stethoscope

    d. The meal and stethoscope, but not the gift certificate

    e. None of the gifts

HIV/AIDS-SPECIFIC ISSUES

29. A 32-year-old pregnant woman comes to your prenatal clinic. She has a history of syphilis and gonorrhea in the past but her VDRL/RPR is negative now. An HIV test is offered as a routine part of her prenatal evaluation as well as because of the history of previous STDs. You explain to her the importance of the test for her baby's well-being. She refuses the test when offered.

    What should you do?

    a. No test; she has the right to refuse.
    b. PCR RNA viral load testing as an alternative.
    c. Consent for HIV testing is not needed in pregnancy because it is to protect the health of the baby.
    d. Add the test to the other routine tests that are to be drawn.
    e. Administer empiric antiretroviral therapy to prevent perinatal transmission.
    f. HIV testing is now part of routine prenatal care and no specific consent is needed.

30. You have a patient who is an HIV-positive physician. He has recently found out that he is HIV-positive. He is very concerned about confidentiality and you are the only one who knows he is HIV-positive. He asks you who you are legally obligated to inform.

    What should you tell him?

    a. His insurance company
    b. State government
    c. His patients
    d. His patients, only if he performs a procedure such as surgery where transmission can occur
    e. No one without his direct written consent
    f. His employer
    g. The hospital human resources department

31. You have an HIV-positive patient in need of drainage of a dental abscess. There is a dentist in your multispecialty group practice. He knows you are an infectious diseases/HIV specialist. Your office manager tells you the dentist and his staff are "scared of your HIV-positive patients" and they don't want to see them.

    What is your response?

    a. This is illegal; the dentist is liable and can be sued.

    b. You contact the medical director and have him instruct the dentist to see the patient.

    c. You prescribe the use of oral antibiotics alone instead.

    d. Refer your patient to another dentist outside of your group practice.

32. You are evaluating a new patient that has come to your clinic for management of his HIV infection. He has high CD4 cells and a low viral load and does not require treatment. He is married and does not practice safe sex with his wife. His wife is unaware of her husband's HIV status.

    What is your duty?

    a. Encourage discussion between the husband and wife and strongly suggest he disclose his HIV status to his wife.

    b. You must keep his HIV status entirely confidential at all times

    c. Have the city Department of Health inform the wife.

    d. Send the wife a letter to come to your office because of an "urgent health issue" and then inform her yourself.

    e. There is no need for partner notification as long as they are practicing safe sex.

33. You have an HIV-positive patient in the office. You ask her if she has informed her partner that she is HIV-positive. She has repeatedly resisted your attempts to have her inform the partner. She is pregnant with his child. The partner is in the waiting room and you have met him many times.

    What should you do?

    a. Inform the partner now.

    b. Respect her confidentiality.

    c. Refer your patient to another physician who is comfortable with her wishes.

    d. Tell the partner to practice safe sex from now on but don't tell him her HIV status

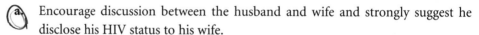

IMPAIRED DRIVERS

34. An 87-year-old man comes to see you for follow-up to a minor concussion sustained a few weeks ago. He was in a minor motor vehicle accident in which his head hit the dashboard but he did not lose consciousness. Your patient has glaucoma and presbycussis. He renewed his driver's license by mail two years ago and the only restriction is that he must wear glasses. You are uncertain whether the patient should be driving.

What should you do?

    a. Inform the patient's family and explain to them that they should not allow the patient to continue driving because it is dangerous for him.

    b. MRI of the brain.

    c. Neurology evaluation.

    d. Start aricept to improve his memory.

     e. Discuss the issue with the patient and encourage him to find alternate methods of transportation.

    f. Remove his license from him.

    g. Mandatory reporting to the police.

INFORMED CONSENT/DECISION-MAKING CAPACITY

35. A 37-year-old man comes to your office for his regular visit. He has seemed severely depressed for some time but refuses to discuss either his feelings or treatment options of any kind. He does not want to use antidepressant medications. His only medications are vitamins. Your relationship with him is excellent but he just won't confront his feelings of depression although he firmly denies suicidal ideation. You prescribe a serotonin reuptake inhibitor for him and tell him that it is a vitamin. Over the next several months his mood markedly improves and he feels much better.

Which of the following most appropriately characterizes your action toward the patient?

    a. Your action is appropriate because it benefited the patient.

    b. Your action is appropriate because there were no side effects.

    c. Your action is not appropriate because you are not a psychiatrist.

    d. Your action is not appropriate because you treated the patient without his consent.

    e. Your action is appropriate because you are sincerely trying to help the patient.

    f. Your action is acceptable as long as you inform the patient now that he is feeling better.

36. A 67-year-old woman is diagnosed with breast cancer. She is fully alert and very specifically both verbally and in writing tells you that she does not want to have surgery on her breast to remove the tumor. She fully understands her condition and treatment options. This is a decision her husband and son both disagree with. Over the next several weeks the patient becomes confused and loses the capacity to understand the details of her medical care. The husband and son now approach you to perform the surgery.

Which of the following is most appropriate?

    a. Refuse to do surgery and follow the original advance directive.

    b. Perform the surgery only if the request is in writing.

    c. Honor the family's request and perform the surgery.

    d. Consult the ethics committee.

    e. Ask the family to seek a court order.

    f. Perform the surgery only if you really believe that it will benefit the patient in the long term.

37. A 52-year-old man with cerebral palsy is being evaluated for screening colonoscopy. He has a mental age of 8 and a second-grade reading level in terms of comprehension. He lives alone and survives on a combination of public assistance and a low-paying part-time job sweeping floors. You have thoroughly explained the procedure to him in terms of risks and benefits. He repeatedly refuses the procedure entirely on the basis of "I just don't want it."

    What should you do?

    a. Perform the procedure.

    b. Seek consent from the family.

    c. Honor his decision and do not do the colonoscopy.

    d. Seek a court order mandating the procedure.

38. Mr. M. consents to a procedure on his left ear. After the patient is anesthetized Dr. W. discovers that the right ear is in greater need of surgery. What should the surgeon do?

    a. Perform the procedure on the right ear if it is clear that it is more necessary.

    b. Wake the patient up and seek consent for a different procedure.

    c. Seek a second opinion from another surgeon and proceed with the more necessary procedure.

    d. Perform the procedure on both ears.

39. A 52-year-old Spanish-speaking woman has arrived for the first day of a clinical trial of chemotherapy for breast cancer. You suddenly remember the need for signing a consent form. You ask a medical student to "get the consent." He walks up to the patient and says in English, "Sign this," and she signs. She completes the trial but her hair falls out and she files suit against you for an improper informed consent.

    Why will this lawsuit be successful?

    a. The risks of the treatment were not explained.

    b. The explanation was not in a language you were sure she could understand.

    c. She experienced harm from the study medication.

    d. Someone who didn't understand the study obtained the consent.

    e. All of the above.

40. An unconscious man is brought to the emergency department for a motor vehicle accident hemorrhaging profusely, hypotensive, and stuporous. You have never met the patient before and no one at your institution knows him. He is wearing a T-shirt that says "Kiss me, I'm a Jehovah's Witness."

    What should you do about the blood transfusion?

    a. Give the blood.
    b. Wait for him to awaken enough to sign consent.
    c. Wait for the family.
    d. Seek a court order.
    e. Give intravenous fluids alone.

41. A 34-year-old man is brought to the emergency department with fever, headache, and a change in mental status leading to significant disorientation. His head CT is normal and he is in need of an urgent lumbar puncture and intravenous antibiotics. He is agitated and is waving off anyone who tries to get near him. Co-workers accompany him. The resident informs you that the patient is pushing away the lumbar puncture needle.

    What should you do?

    a. Sedate the patient with lorazepam and perform the lumbar puncture.
    b. Wait for the family to obtain consent.
    c. Use blood cultures as an alternative.
    d. MRI of the brain.
    e. Ask the co-workers to sign consent.

42. A man is admitted for the management of neutropenia and fever from aplastic anemia. His anemia is severe and his medical care requires blood in addition to antibiotics. He is suffering from a profound delirium from the fever and has lost capacity to understand his problems. His brother is his health-care proxy. The patient is a Jehovah's Witness and is adamantly opposed to transfusion even if he dies, and the brother is not opposed. The patient has clearly told both you and the brother this in the past. The patient's brother believes that the proscription against transfusions is "barbaric and stupid."

What should the patient's brother do?

    a.   Arrange a Jehovah's Witness meeting to discuss the situation.

    b.   Ask their parents to make the decision.

    c.   Ask the doctor to make the decision.

    d.   He should not give consent for the transfusion.

    e.   He should give consent for transfusion.

43. Mr. Sakiewiec is a 32-year-old man with severe mental retardation who has been institutionalized since childhood. He is noncommunicative and has never been able to verbalize his preferences on any decision. His parents are dead and the institution and a court-appointed guardian manages him. He has developed leukemia that is severe and incurable. Chemotherapy involves significant risk and discomfort and only a small chance of prolonging his survival.

What should be done in terms of his medical treatment?

    a.   Proceed with the chemotherapy.

    b.   Confer an "expert panel" to determine therapy.

    c.   Bone marrow transplantation.

    d.   Ask the guardian what is in the best interests of the patient.

44. A 27-year-old pregnant woman presents in her last trimester of pregnancy with severe cephalopelvic disproportion. Her physicians have recommended a caesarian section. She does not want to undergo the surgery. She fully understands the procedure and she is unwilling to suffer the discomfort of surgery. She has been informed that without the C-section her fetus may not survive childbirth.

    What should you do?

    a. Honor her wishes and do not perform the C-section.
    b. Psychiatry evaluation.
    c. Sedate her and perform the surgery.
    d. Obtain a court order to perform the surgery.
    e. Explain the situation to the baby's father and ask him for consent.

45. A 52-year-old man sees you in follow-up after a radical prostatectomy. He had been fully informed about the risk of the procedure such as incontinence and impotence. Neither of these adverse effects occurs. While searching on the Web he finds that there is treatment without surgery involving the implantation of radioactive seeds or pellets in the prostate. He files suit against you because of an improper informed consent.

    What will be the most likely outcome of the suit?

    a. He will lose because there were no adverse effects.
    b. He will lose because all the risks of the surgery were explained to him before he signed consent.
    c. He will lose because radical prostatectomy is a standard procedure.
    d. He will win because you did not inform him of the risks and benefits of alternative therapy to surgery.
    e. He will win because radioactive seeds are the superior form of therapy.

46. A 58-year-old man is out of town on business in New York. He has a myocardial infarction and deteriorates despite thrombolytics and angioplasty. He is intubated and is disoriented and unable to understand his condition. He needs a coronary bypass. His wife is the health-care proxy but she is in another city. You would like her consent in order to perform the surgery because she is the designated surrogate.

    Which of the following is true in this case?

    a. She must come to the hospital to sign consent in person.

    b. The wife must designate a local guardian until her arrival.

    c. You must repeat the angioplasty instead.

    d. Telephone consent is only valid for minor procedures.

    e. Take consent for the bypass over the phone and have a second person witness the telephone consent.

47. Mr. Dorone is a 22-year-old man who sustained a subdural hematoma and a brain contusion in a motor vehicle accident. He needs blood in order to have the necessary lifesaving surgery done. His parents refuse to allow the transfusion based on their religious beliefs.

    What should be done?

    a. Honor the parents' wishes and do not give the blood.

    b. Give the blood.

    c. Wait for a formal hearing with a judge and a court.

48. A 27-year-old Jehovah's Witness is in labor and bleeding heavily. She categorically refuses all transfusions and signs a refusal to consent form indicating that she understands she may die without the blood. When she loses consciousness her husband, who is not a Jehovah's Witness, says to give the blood and he will sign consent.

    What should you tell him?

    a. You will honor his wish if he is the proxy.

    b. You will honor his wish and give the blood.

    c. You will give the blood only if the patient is unconscious.

    d. You cannot give the blood.

KAPLAN MEDICAL

MALPRACTICE

49. A medical resident admits a patient overnight with uncontrolled blood pressure. He means to write an order for the angiotensin receptor blocker Diovan at 10 mg once a day. Because of his sloppy handwriting the nurses and pharmacy administer digoxin at 10 mg a day. This is a drug that is rarely used at a dose above 0.5 mg a day. Three days later, the patient develops a hemodynamically unstable rhythm disorder that the resident very sincerely tries to decipher but is unable to until the patient transfers to the intensive care unit. At this point they discover the overdose of digoxin. The patient and the family never discover the overdose.

Which of the following most accurately describes this situation?

   a. There is no liability for the resident because the overdose was unintentional.

   b. There is no liability for the resident because the pharmacy should have detected the error.

   c. No liability exists because the error is unknown to the patient.

   d. No liability exists because it was an accident.

   e. The resident and hospital are both liable for harm to the patient.

   f. No liability exists because there was no permanent harm to the patient.

50. Which of the following most closely represents the role of risk management in the hospital?

   a. To ensure proper ethical management of patients

   b. To ensure proper clinical care of patients

   c. To act as a patient advocate

   d. To clarify communications from the medical staff to the patient

   e. To minimize the legal risk to the hospital from litigation

51. You explained the risks and benefits of bone marrow transplantation versus chemo-therapy to a woman with leukemia. This was part of an IRB-approved trial. You told her that the transplant has the highest chance of cure of the disease but also the high-est risk of immediate death. She understood what you said and signed the consent for transplantation. She dies as a result of the bone marrow transplant and her husband sues you for wrongful death.

What will be the most likely outcome?

a. He loses the lawsuit because BMT is the standard of care for this patient's age and disease.

b. He wins because he was not informed.

c. He wins because chemotherapy has less risk of death.

d. He loses it because the patient was fully informed about the risks and benefits of both alternatives.

e. He loses because the trial was IRB-approved.

52. A 57-year-old corporate executive comes to the emergency department with an ST segment elevation myocardial infarction. He receives thrombolytics but has persistent chest pain, worsening left ventricular function, and a new S3 gallop. The patient asks you about the risks and benefits of angioplasty. You tell him he could have a hema-toma or a coronary rupture as an adverse effect of the angioplasty balloon. You tell him that the benefit will be that it stops the chest pain. He opts for further medical management without angioplasty because of fear of adverse effects. He dies and his estate sues you.

What will be the most likely outcome?

a. You win because you fully informed him of the adverse effects of the procedure.

b. You win because he refused the treatment offered.

c. You lose because patients cannot refuse lifesaving therapy.

d. You lose because you should have done the angioplasty before the thrombolyt-ics.

e. You lose because you did not inform the patient of the serious consequences of forgoing angioplasty.

53. A 72-year-old woman is admitted to the hospital with gastroenteritis and dehydration. There are no indications in the chart of her having dizziness. She also does not directly inform the nurses of her dizziness. She asks to be brought to the bathroom. She is left alone on the toilet when she becomes lightheaded, faints, and hits her head against a wall sustaining a laceration. The patient and her family subsequently file suit against the hospital for negligence.

    What will be the most likely outcome?

    a. She wins secondary to the negligence of the nurses.

    b. She wins secondary to the negligence of the physicians.

    c. She wins if she has sustained significant brain damage.

    d. She loses because there was no significant injury.

    e. She loses because she did not inform the nurses she was dizzy or lightheaded.

MEDICAL ERRORS

54. A 70-year-old man is admitted to the hospital with endocarditis. At seven days of therapy the antibiotic order expires and you forget to reorder the medication for two days in the middle of a four-week course of intravenous antibiotics. There is no clinical deterioration and the antibiotics are restarted.

    What should you tell the patient?

    a. Tell the patient it was a clerical error.

    b. Because it was not clinically significant you do not have to say anything to the patient.

    c. Apologize and tell the patient that you forgot to reorder the antibiotics, but that he will be all right.

    d. Inform your chief resident but not the patient.

    e. Ask the nurse to tell the patient about the error.

55. You are a resident managing a private patient with cellulitis. The patient has a history of congestive heart failure and a normal EKG. The patient is on digoxin, an ACE inhibitor and a diuretic, but not a beta-blocker. You cannot find a contraindication to the use of beta-blockers either in the chart or in discussion with the patient. You ask the private attending why there is no beta-blocker and he looks at you as if you had anoxic encephalopathy. He says, "I have been in practice for 40 years. Don't you think I know what I am doing? Beta-blockers are dangerous in congestive failure." The patient looks proudly at the attending and says, "I have the smartest doctor in the world."

    What should you do about this disagreement?

    a. Wait for the attending to leave and give the patient a prescription for carvedilol.

    b. Suggest to the patient that he should find another doctor.

    c. Report the physician to the state licensing board.

    d. Do nothing; he is the attending of record.

    e. Bring the disagreement to the chief of service.

    f. Help the patient find a good lawyer and volunteer to testify.

MEDICAL RECORDS

56. A patient of yours has gone to the hospital to obtain a copy of her medical record for her own review. The hospital refuses to release them to her on the grounds that she must provide an adequate reason for wishing to see the records. She has come to see you to ask if this is true and how can she get her records.

    What should you tell her?

    a. You, as the physician, can get the records for yourself to view, but she cannot.

    b. The hospital will give her the records as long as you ask.

    c. She has the right to have her own records as long as she has a legitimate reason.

    d. She has the right to her own records even without giving a reason.

    e. Only another physician, hospital, or insurance company can have free access to her records.

    f. She can have the records as long as she has fully paid her hospital bills.

57. Which of the following most accurately describes the ownership of the medical record?

    a. The record is entirely the property of the patient.

    b. The record is entirely the property of the health-care provider.

    c. The information is the property of the patient and the physical paper or electronic record is the property of the health-care provider.

    d. The information is the property of the health-care provider and the physical paper or electronic record is the property of the patient.

58. A man comes to the emergency department after a stab wound. Your notes document a 500-mL loss of blood. Later that night the patient develops asystole and dies. You find the loss of blood was originally really 3,000 mL, which was not recorded by you.

    What should you do to correct the documentation?

    a. Use correction fluid to eliminate the original note.

    b. Erase the original note.

    c. Remove the original note from the chart.

    d. Write a new note timing and dating it at the same time as the original note.

    e. Write a new note with the current date and time.

MINORS

59. The neighbor of a 14-year-old boy brings him to the emergency department after sustaining a slight laceration to the scalp from head trauma. You evaluate him and determine that suturing of the scalp will be necessary.

    Which of the following is the most accurate?

    a. He is an emancipated minor; the patient can give consent.

    b. The neighbor can give consent.

    c. Wait for the consent of at least one parent.

    d. Wait for the consent of both parents.

    e. Seek a court-appointed legal guardian.

    f. Consent is not necessary in this case.

60. A 15-year-old girl comes to the clinic for dyspareunia and a vaginal discharge. On speculum examination you find she has cervicitis. The pregnancy test is negative. The infection is modest and there is no emergency.

Which of the following is the most appropriate action to take?

a. Ceftriaxone/azithromycin now in a single dose.

b. Make at least a "good faith" effort to notify her parents and treat her.

c. Wait to inform at least one parent.

d. Treat only if the patient agrees to inform her parents.

e. Treat her now and inform the parents later.

61. A 12-year-old boy and his father are involved in a motor vehicle accident that results in a severe hemorrhage requiring an urgent blood transfusion. Both of them are clearly alert and understand that without the blood they may die. They are both Jehovah's Witnesses and are refusing blood transfusion on religious grounds.

What should you do?

a. Honor their wishes; no transfusions for either one.

b. Obtain a court order to transfuse the child.

c. Give blood to the child but not to the father.

d. Psychiatric evaluation.

e. Use intravenous iron in both of them as a blood substitute.

f. Explain the situation to the child and ask him for consent for the transfusion.

62. A 16-year-old female comes to the clinic after missing a period. Her pregnancy test is positive and she wants to start prenatal care with you. She is adamant that you keep the pregnancy confidential from her parents.

What should you tell her?

a. "I will give you the care you need and keep it confidential."

b. "I will not mention it to your parents unless they ask. I can't lie."

c. "I am sorry, but I must tell them."

d. "I will not tell your parents, but I must inform the father of the baby."

KAPLAN) MEDICAL

63. A 12-year-old girl presents with severe right lower-quadrant abdominal pain and marked tenderness and is found to have acute appendicitis. The child is at a sleep-away camp. You are not able to locate her parents. They are not at home and you cannot reach them on the cell phone. The camp counselor and the director of the camp bring in the child.

    What should you do?

    a. Do not do the surgery without parental consent.

    b. Ask the camp counselor or director for consent.

    c. Ask the patient for consent.

    d. Perform the appendectomy.

    e. Give intravenous antibiotics alone.

64. A 16-year-old female comes in for treatment of severe cystic acne with Accutane (isotretinoin). She lives alone and is self-supporting with a job as a waitress. She has been out of her parents' house for a year and pays all her own bills. You have just finished informing her of the potentially severe teratogenicity of isotretinoin. Her acne is severe and she would still like the isotretinoin.

    What should you tell her?

    a. "This medication cannot be taken by women of reproductive age."

    b. "Use benzoyl peroxide topically instead."

    c. "I will give you the isotretinoin if your parents accompany you."

    d. "I will give you the isotretinoin as requested."

    e. "I will treat you with isotretinoin if you have a consent signed by your parents."

PHYSICIAN-ASSISTED SUICIDE AND EUTHANASIA

65. A 65-year-old man comes to see you because he wants your help in committing suicide. The patient has recently been diagnosed with metastatic colon cancer but he is not in pain or nauseated. He found out because of a screening colonoscopy and a subsequent staging evaluation. He denies depression and seems to have a normal mood. He is asking for a prescription or combination of medications that he can take to end his life. He says he will wait for a few weeks or months until he starts to feel weak and then he wants to end his life before he becomes debilitated, bed-bound, or a burden to his family.

Which of the following is most appropriate in this case?

a. Provide the pain medications as appropriate but not the means to end his life.

b. Provide the patient with medications he wants to end his life.

c. Have him undergo psychological screening first.

d. Refer him to a specialist in this area.

e. In-patient psychiatric evaluation for suicidal ideation.

f. Start antidepressants.

66. A 79-year-old man comes to see you for assistance in ending his life. The patient is fully competent and has been suffering from progressively worsening amyotrophic lateral sclerosis for several years. He is not immediately preterminal. Despite this, he finds his quality of life to be unacceptable. More important, he correctly predicts that his level of function will deteriorate over the next several months and that he may become ventilator dependent. He is requesting that you administer a lethal injection in his home. He is not depressed. His family is aware of his desire and they are willing to honor the patient's wishes. You have discussed appropriate palliative care issues.

    What should you tell him?

    a. You tell him that you will honor his wish because he is competent and not depressed.

    b. You tell him that you will honor his wish because his condition will worsen over time.

    c. You agree to his wish because he has a right to a better quality of life.

    d. You tell him that you cannot help him because there is no state law authorizing it.

    e. You tell him that under no circumstances can you participate in euthanasia.

    f. You say that it is okay as long as it happens in Oregon.

PHYSICIAN IMPAIRMENT

67. You are a fourth-year medical student on a subinternship in obstetrics. You notice that the resident has come in with alcohol on his breath and some abnormal behavior. No one except you seems to notice.

    What should you do?

    a. Nothing; you are subordinate to the resident.

    b. Talk to the resident directly alone but don't mention it to the program director.

    c. Tell the dean of students.

    d. Report him to the state licensing board.

    e. Report him to the chairperson or program director of his department.

    f. Immediately inform his patients whom you feel are at risk.

68. You are an attending physician at a university hospital. One of the attendings from another division seems to be having memory difficulty. You have found him twice in the hallway having forgotten where he was going. The residents tell you on the side that they don't rely on him at all because "he forgets everything we say anyway." The chief of service knows but doesn't have enough attendings to fill the yearly schedule so he remains in place supervising both resident performance as well as patient care.

    What should you do?

    a. Nothing; the chief of service already knows.
    b. Talk to him directly.
    c. Tell your division head.
    d. Report him to the state licensing board.

69. You are an attending at a large program in New York. You are out at a bar on Saturday night when you notice one of your residents in the same bar. She is clearly drunk. The resident is sitting behind you, too intoxicated to notice your presence. She is kissing a man who you know is not her husband. You leave before she notices you. The following day you see her at the hospital managing patients and supervising interns. Her behavior and medical management seem completely normal.

    What should you do?

    a. Speak to her directly about her behavior.
    b. Discuss it with her program director or department chair.
    c. Report her to the committee for physician impairment.
    d. Do nothing.

PHYSICIAN/PATIENT RELATIONSHIP

70. A physician in a busy inner-city environment has developed his practice over the years to the point where he no longer needs to solicit new patients. He does not want to expand his hours of work so he decides to limit his practice. He instructs his office staff to begin refusing to accept new patients.

    Which of the following most appropriately describes his action?

    a. It is both legal and ethical.

    b. It is ethically acceptable, but illegal.

    c. He is within his legal rights to refuse patients, but it is considered ethically unacceptable.

    d. It is both illegal and unethical to refuse to accept new patients.

    e. It is ethical as long as he arranges transfer of care to another physician.

71. You have a patient who has recently been diagnosed with myeloma and he is discussing treatment options with you. You are the full-time employee of an outpatient facility run by a managed-care plan and you have recently received written instructions not to bring up subjects such as bone marrow transplantation in myeloma with patients. The reasoning was that they are outrageously expensive and do not cure the disease, although it may extend survival. The data that they extend survival are not entirely conclusive. In addition, in a private meeting with the medical director, you have been told that the expenditures per patient load of care of each of the physicians would be examined yearly to determine which physician would be promoted.

    What do you do?

    a. Fully inform the patient about the risks and benefits of bone marrow transplantation.

    b. Refer your patient to an oncologist to have this discussion.

    c. Transfer the patient to another primary-care provider.

    d. Advise the patient to file suit against the managed care plan.

    e. Give the patient treatment with melphalan or thalidomide.

    f. Inform the patient about bone marrow transplantation if he asks you about it.

72. You have a patient who is a 57-year-old man with a history of HIV who has recently been found to have severe coronary artery disease. He has three vessels with more than 90 percent occlusion and left ventricular dysfunction. He is referred for bypass surgery. The cardiothoracic surgeon at your hospital refuses to operate on your patient because he is scared of touching HIV-positive patients for fear of seroconversion. He is already on a beta-blocker, ACE inhibitor, and aspirin.

    What should you do?

    a. Add calcium channel blockers.

    b. Perform angioplasty and stenting.

    c. Add clopidogrel.

    d. Have his chief of service compel him to do the procedure.

     e. Refer the patient to another cardiothoracic surgeon.

73. A 60-year-old male physician who is an internist has had a female patient for the last 20 years. Both lost their spouses several years ago. They start spending time together outside the office. The female patient wants to begin a sexual/romantic relationship with the physician.

    What should he tell her?

    a. "I can never do that with you, ever."

    b. "We can be social, but not sexual."

    c. "We need the ethics board's approval first."

     d. "I cannot date you and be your doctor—maybe in the future we can date, after you get another doctor."

    e. "Because this is your initiative we can begin dating."

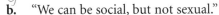

PUBLIC HEALTH AND REPORTING REQUIREMENTS

74. Which of the following does not need to be reported to the health department?

    a. Salmonella

    b. Gonorrhea

    c. Herpes simplex

    d. Tuberculosis

    e. Measles

75. A 38-year-old bus driver is seen in clinic for fever, cough, and sputum with an apical infiltrate as well as sputum positive for acid-fast bacilli. The patient is unwilling to take tuberculosis (TB) medications consistently and his sputum remains positive for TB. Directly observed therapy while in his home has failed. You continue to cajole, discuss, encourage, threaten, educate, advise, and beg him to take the medications but he refuses.

    What should you do?

    a. Nothing, he has a right to autonomy.

    b. Arrest the patient and put him in prison.

    c. Remove the family from the house.

    d. Remove the patient from his job as a bus driver and incarcerate him in a hospital to take medications.

    e. Physically restrain the patient and place a nasogastric tube to give the medications.

76. A 27-year-old man is seen by you after the diagnosis of syphilis. As you are administering his treatment you find he is quite promiscuous. You inform him that you must notify the Department of Health and that his sexual contacts need to be treated. He is extremely embarrassed and asks how they will find out.

What should you tell him?

a. You will notify them yourself but you will not give his name.

b. You will notify them and must let them know he was the contact.

c. You will tell the Department of Health but he himself must tell the contacts.

d. The Department of Health will send a letter or call the contacts and let them know they have a serious health issue. They will test and treat the partners but will not reveal his name.

e. He doesn't have a choice; he has to give the names.

f. Their individual doctors will inform the contacts.

REPRODUCTIVE RIGHTS

77. You are the general internist in a large, multispecialty physician group. The office-based pregnancy test on your patient has just become positive and you estimate the gestational age of the fetus at eight weeks. You are a very deeply religious person in a conservative, midwestern city and you are opposed to abortion because you believe life begins at conception. After extensive discussion about the options, your patient asks to be referred for an abortion.

Which of the following is the most appropriate action?

a. Inform the patient that you are morally opposed to abortion and you cannot make the referral.

b. Terminate your relationship with the patient as her physician.

c. Propose social work/psychological evaluation of the patient.

d. Tell her you will make the referral after a 30-day consideration period in which she may change her mind.

e. Refer the patient for the abortion.

78. A 16-year-old female is in your office because she has just found out she is pregnant. She discusses her options and asks you to refer her for an abortion. She states that her parents do not know she is pregnant and she does not want them to know.

    What should you do?

    a.) Refer her for the abortion without parental notification.
    b. Make a "reasonable effort" to contact the parents, but still refer for the abortion if you cannot contact them.
    c. Do not refer for abortion without parental consent.
    d. Seek a court order declaring her emancipated.
    e. Strongly encourage her to discuss the issue with her parents.

79. A young husband and wife visit your office to discuss methods of contraception. The wife decides that she wants a tubal ligation for sterilization. Her husband is shocked and strongly objects stating that they have no children. His wife is clear that she wants the sterilization and that she wishes to be referred for the procedure.

    What should you do?

    a. Refer for the tubal ligation as requested by the wife.
    b. Refer after a psychological evaluation.
    c. Do not make the referral because she is young.
    d. Do not make the referral because she may change her mind.
    e. Refer only with the husband's consent.

80. A 35-year-old married woman with four children is in your office seeking a termination of an unwanted pregnancy in the first trimester. Later in the day after you give the patient the referral, her husband calls and is very distressed because he does not want the abortion to occur. He very much wants to keep the baby and tells you that he even has a name picked out.

    What should you tell him?

    a. You will try to talk his wife out of the abortion.

    b. You will cancel the procedure immediately.

    c. You say you cannot hold up the termination without a court order.

    d. You cannot prevent the abortion without paternity testing confirming that he is the father.

    e. You say you have an absolute duty to the mother to honor her wishes no matter what his personal feelings are.

81. A 30-year-old woman presents to the clinic during her third trimester. The estimated gestational age of the fetus is 28 weeks and she is seeking an abortion. The patient is generally healthy. An ultrasound of the fetus at 26 weeks and routine genetic testing showed no abnormalities.

    What should you tell the patient?

    a. It's okay; you will go ahead with the abortion.

    b. You will be happy to comply if she can get a court order.

    c. No way, third-trimester abortions are prohibited.

    d. Legally you can only do it if her life is at risk.

    e. No, you can't do it because the fetus is normal.

SPOUSAL ABUSE

82. A 42-year-old man comes to see you for routine management when you inquire about multiple scratches and contusions as well as a black eye. He says his wife routinely abuses him and is "beating me up pretty regularly, doc." He denies hitting his wife. You see him a few weeks later and he has a new version of the same injuries. You are very concerned about his injuries and you tell him that you are planning to report the injuries. He very clearly states that he does not want these injuries reported.

    What do you tell him?

    a. You have no choice but to report the injuries because you are a mandatory reporter.

    b. You will report the injury only with his consent.

    c. You will honor his wish but must report it if there is another episode.

    d. There is no spousal abuse reporting.

    e. You will report it if you find evidence that the wife was really the attacker.

SUICIDE

83. A 68-year-old man attempted suicide by driving his car into a telephone pole with the intentional purpose of ending his life. He was found severely hemorrhaging and in the emergency department he refuses to give his consent for surgery necessary to stop the bleeding. He states that he wants to die. He was recently diagnosed with cancer and refused surgery to remove it. He states that his life had been complete and now, he wishes to end it.

    What should you do about the surgery to stop the bleeding now?

    a. Follow his stated wish and withhold surgery.

    b. Perform the surgery.

    c. Obtain a court order to force the surgery.

    d. Ask the family members for consent.

TORTURE

84. You are a civilian physician and you have been asked to participate in the interrogation of a prisoner suspected of carrying out a terrorist attack. There is very significant evidence to prove his participation in planning subsequent attacks. You have been asked to monitor the patient's oxygen level during a simulated "hanging" and "strangulation" of the patient to determine if supplemental oxygen or intubation is necessary.

    What should you do?

    a. It is ethically permissible to participate.

    b. Participation is permissible only if he has been convicted of the crime.

    c. You can participate if there is a court order.

    d. You must have a release signed by the military prior to your participation.

    e. You cannot participate in the purposeful torture of a prisoner.

85. A group of prisoners is brought to a military hospital in which you work. They are to be screened prior to transfer either to long-term imprisonments or, in some cases, to be released. You notice that several of the patients have burns that look like cigarettes were put out on them as well as several broken bones that have started to heal.

    What should you do?

    a. Report the injuries as signs of possible torture.

    b. Report the injuries only on the patients to be released.

    c. If you are a military physician, you should report the injuries.

    d. If you are a civilian physician, you should report the injuries.

    e. Your only duty is to treat the injuries.

KAPLAN) MEDICAL

WITHHOLDING/WITHDRAWAL OF MEDICAL TREATMENT

86. An elderly patient with multiple medical problems has been admitted to your care in the intensive-care unit. The patient is in a persistent vegetative state secondary to anoxic encephalopathy and has now developed sepsis, hypotension, gastrointestinal bleeding, and respiratory failure requiring intubation. There is no improvement expected in the underlying severe brain damage. Renal failure develops to the point of needing dialysis but you feel the dialysis would be completely futile.

    Which of the following is the most appropriate step in management?

    a. Hemodialysis

    b. Peritoneal dialysis

    c. Renal transplantation

    d. Give albumin

    e. Recommend that dialysis not be performed

87. A 33-year-old female boxer sustains a cervical spine fracture during the welterweight championship match in Las Vegas. She has a fracture of C1 and C2 resulting in paralysis from the neck down and is ventilator dependent. She is fully alert and understands her medical condition. There has been no improvement for the last three months and there is no hope of recovery. Her manager is the health-care proxy. She is frustrated but not depressed and is repeatedly and clearly requesting removal from the ventilator. She understands that she will not survive without the ventilator.

    What should you do?

    a. Remove the ventilator as she requests.

    b. Obtain a court order to continue the ventilator.

    c. Seek family consensus on removing the ventilator.

    d. Seek approval of the health-care proxy.

    e. Sedate the patient and continue the ventilator.

88. A 48-year-old woman has developed stage III non-Hodgkin's lymphoma and needs combination chemotherapy for treatment. Without therapy she has no hope of survival beyond a few weeks or months. With therapy she has an 80 percent chance of complete remission. She understands this entirely but insists that she simply does not want the therapy. There is no evidence of depression.

    Which of the following is the most appropriate action?

    a. Psychiatric evaluation.

    b. Ask the family for their opinion.

    c. Seek a court-appointed guardian.

    d. Honor the patient's wishes.

    e. Offer radiotherapy instead.

    f. Risk management evaluation.

89. An elderly patient with progressive Parkinson's disease comes to see you because of fever, cough, shortness of breath, and sputum production consistent with pneumonia. The patient's Parkinson's disease has been worsening and he has become quite depressed. He has insomnia, early morning waking, and weight loss as well as anhedonia. He is refusing antibiotics and is asking for palliative care only to help him die.

    What should you do?

    a. Psychiatric evaluation.

    b. Sedate the patient.

    c. Comply with the patient's wishes.

    d. Seek the opinion of the family.

    e. Refer to the ethics committee.

    f. Comply with the patient's wishes as long as he is DNR.

90. A 55-year-old man has been admitted to the hospital for worsening of his mental status, poor nutrition and inability to eat when fed. The patient has Creutzfeld-Jakob disease and will not likely improve. Over the last several months the patient has told you repeatedly that he does not want to be "kept alive as a vegetable" with artificial nutrition and hydration by any method. The health-care proxy form specifically states there is to be "no placement of a nasogastric or gastric tube for enteral feeding." The health-care proxy agent is a nurse. The proxy insists that you have a jejunostomy (J-tube) placed for feeding telling you the proxy form only excludes the NG and G-tubes.

    What should you do?

    a. Place the J-tube.

    b. Tell the proxy she needs to get a court order for the J-tube.

    c. Tell the proxy she needs an ethics committee evaluation.

    d. Do not place any form of tube for artificial nutrition or hydration.

    e. Transfer the patient's care to another physician who feels comfortable placing the J-tube.

91. A 35-year-old homosexual man is a victim of a motor vehicle accident in which he sustains head trauma resulting in a large subdural hematoma. His breathing is becoming worse and endotracheal intubation is being considered for mechanical ventilation. His family including his mother as well as his male domestic partner is present. His mother insists on the intubation being performed. The domestic partner is the health-care agent. The agent states unequivocally that the patient stated both verbally and in writing that he wished never to be placed on a "breathing machine for any purpose."

    What should you do?

    a. Honor the proxy and do not intubate.

    b. Honor the mother's wishes and intubate the patient.

    c. Consult the ethics committee.

    d. Neurology evaluation.

    e. Try intubation for 24–48 hours to see if he recovers.

    f. Ask the opinion of the rest of the family.

92. A 75-year-old man is admitted for a myocardial infarction and a stroke that leaves him in a persistent vegetative state. He is a widow, never designated a health-care proxy, and left no written evidence of his wishes for himself. His nephew and daughter want to continue all forms of therapy including artificial nutrition and hydration. His son and the patient's brother want to stop everything. Both parties believe they know the wishes of the patient.

What should you do?

   a. Encourage discussion amongst the family.

   b. You, the physician, make the decision in the best interest of the patient.

   c. Stop all forms of therapy.

   d. Obtain a court order seeking a court-appointed guardian.

93. An 84-year-old woman with severe Alzheimer's disease is admitted to your skilled-nursing facility. She has lost the ability to communicate, is bed-bound, and unable to eat. She did not appoint a proxy and there is no written or clear verbal advance directive of what she wanted for herself. Multiple family members routinely visit her and you are unable to achieve a clear consensus amongst the family of what the patient's wishes were.

What should you do in terms of her care?

   a. Follow the wishes of the eldest child.

   b. Follow what you think is best.

   c. Ask another attending physician's opinion.

   d. Ask the hospital administrator for consent.

   e. Pursue an ethics committee evaluation.

94. A 72-year-old man comes to see you because of severe pain from metastatic prostate cancer to the bones. His pain has become progressively more severe and has not responded to localized radiation, flutamide, or goserilin. In addition, numerous pain medications have failed to achieve an acceptable level of analgesia. He needs more intense pain management with subcutaneous or intravenous opiates. He also has severe COPD and there has been concern about the effect of the opiate medications on the patient's respiratory drive. In other words, the only way to achieve a sufficient amount of pain relief is to use medications that may shorten his life, inadvertently, because of respiratory depression. The patient is fully alert and has the capacity to understand the problem.

Which of the following is the most ethical way to approach his pain management?

a. It is all right as long as he is DNR.

b. It is acceptable as long as the patient understands the risks.

c. It is unacceptable to shorten life with physician-administered medications.

d. Intubate the patient then give the pain medications.

e. Leave him in pain as long as the respiratory drive is not impaired.

f. Offer to end his life with pain medications.

95. A 77-year-old woman is admitted with a stroke that renders the patient dependent on endotracheal intubation and mechanical ventilation. There is no hope of recovery and the patient is unable to communicate. There is no health-care proxy and the patient lacks the capacity to understand her problems. Her husband produces a living will signed by the patient on which is written the statement, "I do not wish to be maintained on a ventilator if there is no hope of recovery." He does not recall ever discussing the subject with his wife.

What should you do?

a. Continue the ventilator.

b. Risk management evaluation.

c. Remove the tube and the ventilator.

d. Seek a court order to remove the ventilator.

e. Ask the rest of the family what they think.

96. An 84-year-old woman is admitted with abdominal pain. On the second hospital day she becomes febrile, severely hypotensive, and tachycardic from an intestinal perforation. The patient is disoriented with no capacity to understand her medical problems. There is no response to antibiotics, fluids, and dopamine over the next 48 hours and there are signs of significant anoxic encephalopathy. Although there is no health-care proxy, the family is in uniform agreement on what the patient would have wanted for herself had she been able to speak for herself.

    Which of the following cannot be stopped at the direction of the family?

    a. Ventilator

    b. Blood tests

    c. Dopamine

    d. Fluid and nutrition

    e. Nothing

97. A 73-year-old man has been brought to a chronic-care facility for long-term ventilator management. The patient has advanced COPD and is unable to be weaned from the ventilator. A tracheostomy has been placed. A nasogastric tube is in place to deliver tube feeding. The patient is fully alert, and understands the situation. He is asking to have the nasogastric tube removed because of discomfort.

    What should you tell him?

    a. "I will get that tube out right away, sir."

    b. "Let's see how much you are able to eat first."

    c. "I will pull it out if you let me put in a gastric tube."

    d. "Let me talk to your family first."

    e. "Do you have a health-care proxy?"

    f. "No way dude, we make the decisions around here, not you."

    g. "Only if you promise not to sue me."

    h. "Are you crazy? Do you think I am going to let MY patient starve to death?"

KAPLAN) MEDICAL

98. A 47-year-old man with end-stage renal failure has asked you to stop his dialysis. The patient fully understands that he will die if he stops dialysis for more than a few days or weeks. He is not depressed and not encephalopathic.

What should you tell him?

a. "I need a court order first."

b. "I am sorry; I don't feel comfortable doing that."

c. "I can't do that. Physician-assisted suicide is not ethical."

d. "I will stop when we get you a kidney transplant."

e. "You will feel better if I sedate you so that you stop disagreeing with me."

f. "Although I disagree with your decision, I will stop the dialysis."

g. "I cannot do that. We already started dialysis. Now we have to continue."

h. "Not until you pay your bill."

99. A 92-year-old man with Alzheimer's disease has been admitted to the hospital with aspiration pneumonia. He is on a ventilator and has a nasogastric tube in place. He does not have the capacity to understand his medial condition. You find a living will in an old chart that says "No heroic measures," "I want to be DNR," and "I wish to be kept comfortable." There is no proxy and there is no family available with whom you can discuss the matter. He has no private physician with whom you can discuss the case.

What should you do regarding the ventilator and tube feeding?

a. Continue both for now.

b. Remove the ventilator and the tube feeding.

c. Remove the nasogastric tube but continue the ventilator.

d. Seek a court-appointed guardian.

e. Decide what you think is best for the patient.

100. Which of the following best approximates the role of the health-care proxy?

    a. To explain the physician's plan to the family

    b. To convey the wishes of the family to the medical team

    c. To communicate and carry out the wishes of the patient

    d. To make decisions based on what he or she genuinely believes is the best interests of the patient

    e. To carry out the financial decisions of the patient when he or she loses the capacity to speak

101. A 34-year-old woman with three children presents pregnant at 20 weeks of gestational age with anemia and severe gastrointestinal bleeding requiring transfusion to save her life. She is a Jehovah's Witness and she is refusing blood transfusion.

What should you do?

    a. Honor her wishes; no transfusion.

    b. No transfusion now, but the transfusion is mandatory after the second trimester when the fetus is a potentially viable baby.

    c. Transfuse the patient.

    d. Seek a court order mandating the transfusion.

    e. Get consent of the father of the baby.

KAPLAN MEDICAL

102. Mr. Barber is a 58-year-old man who has a cardiac arrest after surgery. He suffers permanent brain damage from anoxic encephalopathy. He is in a permanent vegetative state and ventilator dependent. His wife and eight children are present in the hospital and request in writing for the ventilator to be stopped. After its removal he continues to breath. They are asking for the intravenous lines to be removed and all blood testing to be stopped. They agree that this was his wish for himself. He did not leave a written advance directive such as a living will but he clearly told his family, "I don't want to be a vegetable." He never designated a health-care proxy.

What should you do?

a. Refer the case to the ethics committee.

b. Obtain a court order.

c. Refuse; you cannot ethically do this.

d. Transfer the care of the patient to another physician.

e. Remove the IV lines and stop blood draws as they wish.

f. You can withhold additional new treatments and tests, but you cannot stop those already started.

Answers and Explanations

No Need for Further Studies When Brain Dead

1. **(a) Remove the ventilator.**

The patient meets the criteria for brain death. These are: negative corneal reflex, no nystagmus in response to caloric stimulation of the tympanic membranes, negative pupilary and oculocephalic reflexes, and the absence of spontaneous respiration when the ventilator is held. If there are no brainstem reflexes and the patient will not spontaneously breathe, then the patient is brain dead. There is no hope of recovery in this circumstance. An EEG is not necessary because the clinical presentation is clearly consistent with brain death. Brain death is the legal definition of death in the United States. Although the heart has continued to beat, it is the same as taking the heart out of the chest and seeing it beat in a specimen pan simply because of the automaticity of the heart's intrinsic conduction pathway. When a patient is brain dead, you do not need to seek court or ethics committee approval prior to stopping all therapy. When a patient is brain dead, do NOT place a nasogastric tube for feeding or hydrate the patient. The brain-dead patient is dead. This would be as illogical as placing a naso-gastric feeding tube in a cadaver on the autopsy table.

Remember, although you have legal right to turn off the ventilator immediately on a person who is brain dead, you should talk to the family first. If there is an answer that says "discuss," "conference," or any other words indicating that you want to always achieve consensus first, then that is the answer. The boards would greatly prefer you discuss the matter with the patient's family first, prior to removing the endotracheal tube.

Mandatory Reporting

2. (h) **Report the family to child protective services.**

    Although, in general, it is better to address issues directly with patients and their families, this is not the case when you strongly suspect child abuse. Reporting of child abuse is mandatory even based on suspicion alone. Although it is frightening to be confrontational with the family, the caregiver is legally protected even if there turns out to be no abuse as long as the report was made honestly and without malice. You do not have the authority to remove the child from the custody of the parents. Only child protective services or the courts can do that. The police would be appropriate for an assault happening at that exact moment, but the police are not appropriate to investigate child abuse. When you have a suspicion of child abuse, it doesn't matter what the parents say. That is why talking directly to the mother or father is incorrect. When you suspect abuse, even if the family denies it, you must still report.

Privacy of Health-Care Information in the Workplace

3. (c) **Inform him that you are not at liberty to give details regarding the patient without the patient's permission.**

    Confidentiality is a fundamental right of all patients. As part of maintaining the patient's autonomy in revealing information only to those they wish to be informed of their condition you must refuse to release any specific information of the patient's medical history or current medical problems without direct permission from the patient. Respect this right even if the person asking is, indeed, a co-worker—or even their superior. You have no idea if medical information may be used to discriminate against the patient. Separate from this, third parties have no automatic right to a patient's medical information unless they are directly involved in the care of the patient. This would hold true even if the person seeking information is a health-care worker if they are not directly involved in the care of the patient. Have the patient—not the person requesting the information—sign the consent form for release of information confirming that they are giving you permission to release information.

4. **(d) Tell them you cannot show them the chart unless there is a signed release from the patient.**

You cannot release a patient's medical records unless there is a clear, signed release from the patient or there is a court order. This is true no matter who is asking. If the federal agents have a court order for the records then they have a right to the information. A court order, warrant, or subpoena can be used by the judicial system to violate confidentiality if the judicial system sanctions the violation. Although the medical record as a physical object is the property of the physician or health-care facility, the information is the property of the patient. In a sense, the information is like a person's house. No one has the right to enter your home without either your permission or a court order allowing the investigation. This is also true even if the people requesting it are law enforcement agents. We all have a constitutional right against illegal search and seizure of our property.

Breaking Confidentiality to Prevent Injury to Others

5. **(e) Inform both the patient's boss as well as law enforcement of the threat.**

A patient's right to confidentiality ends where another person's right to safety begins. Your duty to protect the life of the person at risk is more important than keeping the patient's medical information confidential. You must see that the person at risk is duly warned. If law enforcement is informed and the potential victim is not informed then you are held liable if there is injury to the victim.

Duty to Inform the Patient First; Withholding Information from the Patient

6. **(d) You tell them that you are obligated to inform the patient of all the findings.**

Your first duty is to keep the patient fully informed about her health care. Unless there is significant evidence of possible psychological harm to a patient, you have an absolute duty to the patient first, not the family. One of the only examples of possible psychological harm to a patient would be an actively suicidal person who was given significant bad news.

The motives of the family members are irrelevant. Whether they are kind and loving or vindictive and evil makes no difference. This is true whether their request to withhold information is in writing or is from the hospital ethics committee. In this case, the ethics committee is not necessary because there is no substantive question of the right action to inform the patient first. The health-care proxy's opinion and participation are only mandated if the patient loses decision-making capacity. If the patient has decision-making capacity, the health-care proxy's opinion is not different from anyone else's.

Breaking Confidentiality to Inform Others of Genetic Diseases

7. (e) **Inform the patient's ex-wife of the risk to the children.**

The patient's right to confidentiality ends where it comes into conflict with the safety of other people. The right to confidentiality is extremely strong, but it is not universal and absolute. In this case, the children of the patient have a right to know whether their lives will be cut short by the disease of familial adenomatous polyposis (FAP) and colon cancer. The most important element is that screening for polyps should begin at the age of 12 with screening sigmoidoscopy every year. Colectomy needs to be done if polyps are found. Hence, in FAP there is a very specific intervention that can prevent colon cancer and a very specific screening that can be done. In addition, the mother has a right to know whether her children will become ill and how to plan for that. If a child falls and breaks his leg, one parent cannot claim confidentiality as a reason to withhold this critical health information from the other parent. As a part of divorce, the stipulation that each parent must inform the other parent of health-care issues for the children as they arise is a standard part of the agreement. Although, in this case, the health-care issue involves the private health of one parent, the issue is still pertinent to the other parent as the caregiver of the children.

The right to one person's to privacy is not as important as the right of another person to safety. This is established standard and does not require a court order. You will have more liability from the mother of the children if she is NOT informed than from violating the confidentiality of the patient to inform. She can successfully pursue a legal action stating you, the physician, did not inform her that her children were at risk of the "injury" of the genetic disease.

The health department does not do notification for genetic diseases. The health department notifies partners and the population at risk of transmissible diseases such as tuberculosis, HIV, STDs, and food- or water-borne diseases.

Immigration Status Confidential

8. (a) **"Don't worry, the Department of Health does not ask for or report immigration status."**

As a physician our ethical duty is to provide medical care to patients. Physicians have no duty to report immigration status. Neither physicians nor the Department of Health act as information services to report people's immigration status to the government. There is no mandatory reporting of immigration status to the government either before, during, or after the treatment of tuberculosis. Incarceration to take TB medications in active tuberculosis may occur for a noncompliant patient, but they do not specifically face deportation for health reasons. Actually, impaired health is one of the grantable reasons for asylum. Mandatory reporting of immigration status would be a direct impairment of the physician/patient relationship.

Sperm/Egg/Embryo Donation

9. (c) **It is legal to sell both the sperm and eggs but not the embryos.**

The patient can sell and donate unfertilized gametes such as sperm and eggs. Both sperm and eggs are considered equal. A fertilized gamete (or embryo) can also be donated. However, it is currently illegal to sell embryos.

Who Asks for Donation Consent

10. **(e) Organ-donor network**

The rules concerning organ donation are quite specific that the medical team taking care of the patient must not be the ones asking for the donation of organs. This is a conflict of interest. It pits the family's perception of the physician as caregiver against the impression that the medical staff just wants the organs. There can also be significant amounts of irrational thinking associated with grief such as the family thinking you only want to turn off the ventilator so you can harvest the organs. The medical team must stay clearly in the role of the people trying to preserve the life of the patient. The other most practical reason for the organ-donor network to ask is that their chance of successfully obtaining consent is far, far in excess of physicians who ask. The organ-donor network doing the asking both preserves the ethical integrity of the medical team in the eyes of the family as well as markedly increasing the supply of viable organs available for donation.

Payment for Organ Donation Is Unacceptable

11. **(e) Reimbursement for cost of travel and lodging for the donation is acceptable, but profiting from the donation is unacceptable.**

There is an enormous shortage of acceptable organs for donation. As such, cash payment would favor the organs going to the person who was the wealthiest, not the person with the best match or greatest need for the organ. The organs must be uniformly and fairly distributed. If selling organs is considered unethical in the United States, then it is unethical to participate in a cash-for-organ practice anywhere. As physicians we cannot have separate domestic and international ethical systems.

Family Refusal Can Overrule the Organ-Donor Card

12. (e) **Honor the wishes of the family; no donation.**

Although the organ-donor card indicates the patient's wish to donate his organs, it is still unacceptable to harvest organs against the direct wish of the family. If we were to overrule the family, then there would be no point in asking them to consent. Why ask consent for donation, if we would take the organs anyway even if they said no? The organ-donor card is an indication of the patient's wishes but it is not fully binding.

DNR Does Not Limit Other Forms of Treatment

13. (c) **Go ahead with the dialysis; ignore the DNR order.**

A "Do-Not-Resuscitate" (DNR) order is very specifically defined as refraining from cardiopulmonary resuscitative efforts such as chest compressions, antiarrhythmic medications such as amiodarone or lidocaine, and electrical cardioversion in the event of the patient's cardiopulmonary arrest. A DNR order has nothing to do with any of the other forms of care that the patient is receiving. A DNR order has no impact on the use of dialysis. You should pretend that the DNR order does not exist when evaluating for dialysis. Hyperkalemia is life threatening. It is illogical to use an inferior therapy such as kayexalate for the long-term management of the hyperkalemia of renal failure if dialysis is indicated. This patient is awake, alert, and able to understand his or her own medical problems. The patient's family is not relevant in terms of the decision-making pathway if the patient has the capacity to understand his or her own medical problems.

DNR Does Not Preclude ICU Management

14. **(c) Transfer to the ICU as needed; okay to be DNR in the ICU.**

A "Do Not Resuscitate" or DNR order means no cardiopulmonary resuscitative efforts in the event that the patient dies. There is to no other automatic limitation in therapy besides this. DNR orders are often confused with generalized withholding of care such as transfusion or ICU management. DNR orders are not the same as stopping the active management of the patient. DNR orders do not automatically mean that the patient is immediately terminal or that there is an automatic assumption of palliative care only.

15. **(e) DNR does not preclude surgery; proceed with the appendectomy.**

DNR is not meant to be a generalized limitation on all forms of therapy. You can still intubate patients even if they are DNR. No additional forms of consent are required even if they are DNR. DNR just means you are taking death as the endpoint of giving treatment. In the event of cardiopulmonary arrest do not give the additional therapy of cardiopulmonary resuscitation, defibrillation, and chest compressions. DNR is not a general equivalent for withholding any other forms of therapy except these.

Reporting of Elder Abuse Mandatory

16. **(f) Report the grandson-in-law's abuse to adult protective service.**

Elder abuse is common and you have the right to report the abuse over the objections of the patient in the majority of states. The reporting requirements for elder abuse are like child abuse except that they are not uniformly mandatory in all states. Although the legal requirements are not identical in all states, the ethical requirement of physicians to report abuse is clear and uncompromising. The reporting of elder abuse does not depend on the wishes of the patient. With the elderly you often have a competent adult who is simply frail or impaired in some other way. Although the patient may see the loss of the care of the family as a worse problem than their injuries, you must act to protect the patient from an environment that might kill her. You cannot speak to the grandson or notify the police without the patient's approval. Home health aids are there to clean, cook, dress, and otherwise maintain the patient's needs, but they are not security personnel.

Direct Physician Participation Not Ethical

17. **(d) "I am sorry; I cannot participate in the execution at all as a physician."**

The ethical guideline of the American Medical Association and the American College of Physicians are expressly clear that a physician cannot participate in "any action which would directly cause the death of the condemned or assist another individual to directly cause the death of the condemned." This includes starting the intravenous line, mixing the medications, formulating the medications, administering the medication, and even giving technical advice. In fact, it is unethical even to be observing an execution in your capacity as a physician because it gives the suggestion of your acquiescence to the procedure. It is not ethically permissible to certify the death unless it has already been determined by another person. The primary role of the physician in terms of beneficence (doing good to others) and nonmaleficence (not doing harm) are completely incompatible with participating in executions. If you are the physician in a prison your physician/patient relationship cannot simultaneously contain both the role of the caregiver and the executioner's facilitator depending on the day of the week. It is ethically permissible to give anxiolytic medications prior to the day of execution to relieve the suffering of the person condemned.

KAPLAN MEDICAL

Necessity of Informed Consent

18. **(b) Informed consent is required to participate.**

All clinical trials require informed consent. Experimental subjects have an absolute right to know that they are participating in a trial. This is true even if the medication studied had only benefit and no adverse effect. You would still need informed consent. As a principle of autonomy, you do not have the right to do something for someone or to someone without her consent, even if it helps you. In this sense, I could not give you money as a gift without your consent. The design of the institutional review board (IRB) is to assure the ethical integrity of all clinical trials at an institution or facility. An IRB is an independent board of reviewers who must not have any direct gain or harm from the implementation of the trial in order to assure objectivity. All human experiments require the approval of the IRB.

Hence, if I designed a trial comparing whether me giving you $50 or $100 as a tax-free gift made you happier, I would still need to get IRB approval and you would have to sign an informed consent.

Prisoner Participation in Experimentation

19. **(d) Their rights are identical to those of a nonprisoner.**

Prisoners have the right to participate in clinical research trials. They are also entitled to monetary compensation for their participation. Participation cannot be used as a criterion for shortening their prison sentence. Essentially, prisoners have all the same rights in terms of their participation in clinical research as nonprisoners. This also includes the right to refuse participation. It is not unethical for them to participate. The ethical difficulties begin when the power of choice and informed consent are removed from the prisoner. Incarceration does not reduce the prisoner to the subhuman, animal-like status of unfair treatment or not having the right to refuse participation. Clinical trials that occur in a prison must undergo the same review process by an institutional review board (IRB) as those occurring outside the prison. You cannot force someone into research just because he is a prisoner. You cannot coerce them into participating by suggesting it will shorten the prison sentence.

Disclosing Financial Affiliations at the Time of Publication

20. **(d)** **There are no restrictions on your authorship as long as you disclose the financial affiliation.**

There is no automatic ethical difficulty with industry sponsorship of clinical trials and experimentation. Financial support from a company does not eliminate you as an author as long as you disclose all of your financial affiliations with the company. The absolute requirement to reveal financial or business affiliations at the time of publication is necessary for all the authors. This is true even if the data are accurate and unbiased. You must reveal grant support for your trial even if the payments are made to a third party such as the hospital or medical school. You may still have been influenced to alter the outcome even if you have not personally received the payments directly into you own bank account. The key issue in terms of research and publications is not whether you or your institution took money from companies but revealing the financial connections between the authors and the company.

Role of the IRB

21. **(c)** **Ensure the ethical and humane treatment of human subjects in experimentation**

The institutional review board (IRB) reviews all experimental trials to make sure that the treatment of the subjects is fair and humane. Part of this responsibility is to make sure there is adequate informed consent and that the asked question is a valid question. In other words, the IRB will make sure that the placebo end of the trial does not withhold clearly beneficial therapy simply to collect data. The IRB makes sure that all human subjects understand precisely what they are agreeing to participate in. The IRB makes sure that there is sufficient monitoring of the study so that if a treatment is found definitely harmful or helpful then the trial stops in order to switch the subjects into the more beneficial arm of it, once the point has been proven.

IRBs developed out of the experience of the Nazi war crimes tribunal at Nuremburg in which it became clear that experimentation was performed on humans without their consent and without concern for safety. The IRB ensures that the patient never suffers purposeful harm simply to answer a scientific question. In short, the function of the IRB is to ensure that the care of the subject in the trial is more important than the collection of data. You cannot use an unethical means to achieve an ethical end.

Employer Wants Mandatory Genetic Testing of Workers

22. **(d) Ask the patient if she wants the test performed and the results reported.**

Employers do not have a right to the confidential health-care information of patients. You may perform and report certain tests to the employer at the request of the patient. In addition, genetic testing is, as of yet, of unproven value. It is not yet clear what to do with the results of these tests in terms of their impact on the standard management of patients. A positive test for the APC gene does not mean the patient will get cancer of the colon. A negative test does not mean that the patient will not get cancer. A negative test is insufficiently sensitive to rule out cancer. The negative predictive value is insufficient to rule out cancer. The only thing that is clear about the ethics of the genetic testing for cancer is that we wish to prevent discrimination and there can be no mandatory reporting of genetic information.

Genetic Information Privacy

23. **(d) Refuse to provide the information to the employer.**

The employer has no right to the genetic information of a patient. Cancer is not transmissible to fellow employees. None of the genetic tests have an impact on job performance or job safety, which are the only forms of information that an employer has a claim to.

Gifts from Industry

24. (c) **Do not accept the money, but the dinner and the lecture are ethically acceptable.**

Drug companies constantly surround physicians in an attempt to influence prescribing patterns. It is ethically acceptable to participate in educational activities sponsored by the pharmaceutical industry. Modest meals are also ethically acceptable. Although the speaker may accept a cash honorarium for preparing and giving the lecture, it is not ethically acceptable for members of the audience to accept direct monetary payment for participating. Hence, it is ethically acceptable to attend the lecture and the meal, but not to accept a check for cash for the participants.

Honoraria from Industry

25. (d) **It is permissible to take the money as long as you disclose any other financial or business connection with this or any other company.**

Industry sponsorship of the speakers in medical education is acceptable as long as there is no expectation of the company controlling or influencing the content of the presentation. In other words, you are not allowed to simply be an advertisement for the company pretending to be giving an objective presentation of medical data. Speakers have a mandatory responsibility to disclose all financial participation with industry. This allows the audience to judge for itself whether there is undue influence from industry altering the content of the talk in favor of a particular product. There is no requirement to donate all speakers' fees to charity. There is no requirement for prior review of a presentation to an independent monitoring board for content.

Inappropriate Gifts from Patients

26. (b) **"Thank you very much, but I cannot accept."**

You cannot accept gifts from patients who are clearly having evidence of an acute psychiatric disturbance. Even if the patient is not ill enough to qualify as incompetent, gifts from patients must be truly objective and clean in a way that there can be no question of acute emotional duress leading to the gift.

Acceptable Gifts from Patients

27. **(b) Accept the gift.**

Small gifts from patients of limited value are ethically acceptable. Food, plants, and small articles of clothing such as a scarf are all acceptable. Refusing such signs of gratitude would be hurtful to the doctor/patient relationship if they are a sign of the good relationship with you. Gifts can never be tied to a specific expectation of care such as a particular prescription or the successful completion of paperwork such as disability forms. There is no reporting or disclosure requirement for small gifts of nominal value.

Acceptable Gifts from Industry

28. **(a) All the gifts**

Acceptable gifts from industry are never tied to particular practice patterns, specific drug prescribing habits, or any expectation of practice behavior chance particular to a specific product. Industry may sponsor educational experiences as long as they are not restricting the content in any way. Besides modest meals, the other forms of acceptable gifts are those with direct educational or medical value that enhance the care of patients. Direct monetary payments for simple participation are not acceptable. In this case, the gift of a stethoscope will only enhance patient care. The gift certificate is acceptable because it is to a medical school bookstore. A gift certificate to a department store would not be acceptable. The value of gifts should generally be small. Gifts should not be geared merely to entertainment. Tickets to concerts or sporting events are not acceptable. Pens, notepads, and small pieces of medical equipment such as a stethoscope or reflex hammer are acceptable.

Pregnancy, Right to Refuse Testing

29. (a) **No test; she has the right to refuse.**

Patients cannot be tested for HIV against their specific refusal. This is true even in the case of a pregnant woman when the baby's health is at stake. In fact, HIV testing requires an additional layer of consent even though it is only a blood test. We recognize that invasive, potentially complicated procedures such as surgery and endoscopy need additional consent because of the risk of death and morbidity associated with these procedures. In general, blood testing for chemistry or hematology does not need a specific, additional consent beyond general hospital consent. There is a low threshold for accepting that there is implied consent on the basis of the patient's presence in the hospital or office. This is not true in the case of the HIV test. There is no such thing as an "implied" consent for HIV testing. Even though the baby has as much as a 30 percent risk of getting the virus from the mother, the mother cannot be treated against her will. The reasoning is the same. The woman's right to choose the management of her own body outweighs the right of the fetus. An undelivered fetus is not endowed with the power of an individual identity as a "person" in the legal sense. This is the same reasoning as a pregnant woman having the right to refuse a Caesarian section even if the life of the fetus is at risk.

HIV-Positive Caregivers, No Mandate to Inform Patients

30. (e) **No one without his direct written consent**

Patients with HIV have a right to privacy as long as they are not putting others at risk. You have no mandatory obligation to inform the state, his insurance, or his employer. You and the patient do not have a mandatory obligation to inform his patients of his HIV status even if he is a surgeon. This is because an HIV-positive physician poses no significant risk of transmission to a patient. Universal precautions are supposed to prevail in order to prevent transmission. Every patient requires management as if he were HIV-positive in order to interrupt transmission. This is the meaning of "universal" precautions.

There is no implied consent in terms of HIV. It must be expressed in writing. Health-care workers are at risk of HIV from accidental transmission from HIV-positive patients. Yet, there is no requirement that all patients be tested in order to prevent transmission to the health-care worker. All patient blood and body fluids are to be treated as if they were HIV-positive. If the automatic right to know the HIV status of the patient does not exist, then the patient does not automatically have the right to know the HIV status of the physician. It works both ways.

Dentist Refusal to Treat HIV-Positive Patients

31.   (d) **Refer your patient to another dentist outside of your group practice.**

It is unethical for a physician or other health-care worker to decline seeing any particular group of patients based only on a specific disease unless they are being asked to manage a disease that is beyond their area of expertise. Although refusing to see HIV-positive patients is unethical, it is not illegal. You cannot force the dentist to take on a patient without his consent. The medical director cannot do that either. The doctor/patient relationship must be entered in a voluntary way on both sides. You cannot force a doctor to see a patient anymore than a patient can be forced to see a particular physician. Oral antibiotics alone are insufficient for a patient who needs a surgical drainage. The boards often mix an ethical issue with a concrete medical alternative to see if you would pick an inadequate therapy rather than make a decision in an ethical dilemma.

Partner Notification

32. **(a) Encourage discussion between the husband and wife and strongly suggest he disclose his HIV status to his wife.**

    You have a duty both to protect the privacy of your patient as well as to protect the health of innocent third parties. If your patient is practicing unprotected sex with his partner or is sharing needles, he should be strongly encouraged to notify the partner. If this does not happen, you are legally protected to reveal the HIV status of a patient if you believe that person is endangering the life of another person. When partner notification does occur, it is usually the responsibility of the Department of Health. It is the health department that should send the letter to the partners notifying them of the "urgent health issue."

33. **(a) Inform the partner now.**

    You have full legal protection if you inform the partner. The safety of an innocent person is always more important that privacy. You are not legally mandated to inform the partner directly but you are protected if you do. You have no liability in breaking confidentiality for this purpose. You definitely are liable if the patient's partner seroconverts and you did not tell him he was at risk even though you knew. This is a version of the Tarasof case in psychiatry (*Tarasof v. Regents of the State of California*, 17 Cal3d 424 [1976]). If a mentally ill patient discloses to you in confidence that he is planning to injure someone, you have an absolute mandate to inform both law enforcement as well as the person at risk. If you know that harm may occur, but you do nothing, then you are liable. If partner notification is going to occur, you must inform the patient that you will inform her partner.

Mandatory Reporting Is Not National

34. **(e) Discuss the issue with the patient and encourage him to find alternate methods of transportation.**

The laws concerning the impaired driver are not universal between states except for drunk driving. There is no national law guiding physician reporting of an impaired driver for reasons of age, cognitive impairment such as Alzheimer's, or neurological diseases such as multiple sclerosis or Parkinson disease. A few states require mandatory reporting to the Department of Motor Vehicles in order to restrict or remove a driver's license. Most do not. Some states offer protection for physicians in case the report is not honored. Most do not. The rates of motor vehicle accidents remained stable in older patients until the age of 70 when there is a slight rise. However, the highest rate of motor vehicle accidents in all age groups is in those above 85. This group of the very old exceeds even teenagers in terms of the rate of motor vehicle accidents. Because the standards for reporting of the impaired driver varies based on the state, there can be no question where the correct answer is either to report or not to report because this is a national examination. All that can be universally agreed upon is that you should encourage a potentially impaired driver at any age to seek alternate forms of transportation or to have someone else drive.

Misuse of Beneficence

35. **(d) Your action is not appropriate because you treated the patient without his consent.**

A patient must give consent to any test or treatment performed upon him as long as the patient has the capacity to decide. Physicians are not acting ethically when they treat a patient without his consent even if it benefits the patient. It is very difficult for some people to accept that goodwill and sincerity are not sufficient to override the absolute necessity for informed consent. This is true even if you are right in the sense that the treatment will help the patient and that only the patient will benefit from the procedure or treatment. This is true even if payment is not received. Autonomy of the individual outweighs beneficence, which is the desire to do good. This is the physician's desire to treat the patient. Another way of saying it is: I have a right to be sick and miserable if that is what I want.

Decisions Made While Competent Remain Valid When Incompetent

36. (a) **Refuse to do surgery and follow the original advance directive.**

The patient in this question gave a clear advance directive while she still had decision-making capacity. This must be followed. This case is especially clear because it states there is both a clear verbal as well as written advance directive. Cases in which there is no clear advance directive are much harder. It does not matter if the family's request is in writing. The case would be considered too straightforward to warrant the intervention of an ethics committee. Even if the ethics committee for some reason recommended the surgery, you would still have to refuse because your duty is to follow the patient's wishes, no one else's. You cannot refuse a decision made while competent simply because the patient later becomes incompetent. If this were not so, then all wills would be invalid. A person's will is a form of advance directive for their property after they become unable to speak for themselves directly.

Limitation on Determination of Incompetence

37. (c) **Honor his decision and do not do the colonoscopy.**

Just because a patient may be incompetent in certain areas of his life does not mean that he is not able to consent for medical procedures. The patient described has a severe and permanent cognitive impairment; however, he is still able to refuse the procedure. A patient can be considered incompetent for financial issues but still have the ability to make medical decisions. It would not be advisable to recommend routine medical procedures against the will of the patient. This would mean literally forcing him into the endoscopy through restraints or sedation. Incompetence in one area does not mean total incompetence. The court recognizes a much lower standard of cognitive ability to reliably consent or refuse procedures compared with financial decisions. It is easier to be declared incompetent for financial decisions than it is for medical decisions.

Consent Is Specific to Each Individual Procedure

38. (b) Wake the patient up and seek consent for a different procedure.

You must obtain informed consent by specific procedure. Consent for another procedure or clear medical necessity cannot infer consent for another procedure. Neither the medical necessity of the procedure, the seriousness of the condition, nor the assumption that any reasonable person would consent is sufficient to assume that consent is given. The patient is not aware of his surroundings and condition because of the sedation. You cannot have an "informed consent" without waking up and informing the patient. Another example would be a blood transfusion in a Jehovah's Witness. If, during a procedure, a clear but unexpected necessity for blood transfusion arises, you must wake the patient up and ask about the patient's wishes to have or not have blood. The consent or refusal must be informed. You cannot say that because of the necessity or sedation, that you should just give the blood. On the other hand, just because a patient is a Jehovah's Witness, you cannot assume that he will refuse the blood. A refusal must be informed as well. The patient could, after all, be a Jehovah's Witness who does not agree with that religion's teaching on blood. Each procedure must undergo an individual consent process.

Invalid Consent Because of Language and the Wrong Person Obtaining It

39. (e) All of the above.

For consent to be valid, the person who thoroughly understands the procedure must explain the risks of it in a language the patient understands. The hospital is required to provide translators to accomplish this end.

Consent Is Implied in Emergencies

40. **(a) Give the blood.**

In an emergency, unless there is an extremely clear advance directive, there is implied consent to procedures. This patient is not conscious to make a decision. He cannot be fully informed to make a choice. There is no advance directive, proxy, living will, or family available there to be the "substitute" for his judgment. Hence, we must make a decision in the best interests of the patient. A shirt is not a sufficient advance directive. You cannot document that he knows the risks of deferring therapy, which, in this case, is death. Even if he was a Jehovah's Witness, you cannot be certain he would refuse the blood. You cannot say, "Well every other Jehovah's Witness refuses blood, so would he." The refusal must be individual. He, this individual patient, must specifically say he doesn't want the blood in the specific situation.

Otherwise it is like going to a restaurant where all the residents always order pizza. You walk into the restaurant and you are a resident. Should the restaurant automatically serve you pizza? Maybe you want chicken. Shouldn't they ask you what you want? How would you feel if you have on a shirt that says, "Kiss me, I'm a resident" and the waiter brings you pizza saying, "Well, everyone else in your group eats pizza." You must get individual informed consent or refusal, maybe the patient will consent, and maybe he will not. A shirt is not sufficient evidence of a choice of food or blood transfusion.

Emergency Procedure in an Adult Lacking Capacity

41. **(a) Sedate the patient with lorazepam and perform the lumbar puncture.**

The patient described is not able to give informed consent for the procedure nor is he able to make an informed refusal of the procedure. He does not have the capacity to understand his medical condition and the consequences of deferring the lumbar puncture or the antibiotics. There is no proxy or family member available to give consent for the procedure and to substitute for his own judgment. In other words, what would the patient want for himself should he be able to make decisions for himself. The co-worker does not count as a person who can give consent. A blood culture alone or an MRI is insufficient as a diagnostic test to manage meningitis adequately. You cannot wait for the family in a case like this.

If a patient has an urgent, life-threatening, dangerous, or even severely painful medical condition, and the patient is not competent and has no family or proxy available, then the medical staff can do what they feel is necessary to protect the patient without a specific signed consent. You would be more at fault for withholding therapy in this patient than you would to do the lumbar puncture. Acting in his best interests outweighs a formal consent that you cannot immediately obtain.

Substituted Judgment When the Proxy Disagrees with the Patient

42. **(d) He should not give consent for the transfusion.**

The purpose of a health-care proxy is to carry out the wishes of the patient in the event that the patient becomes unable to make decisions for himself. The key issue here is "the wishes of the patient." The proxy is not a person who is just to give his own opinion of what he (the proxy) thinks is best for the patient, if the patient's clear wishes are known. The proxy or health-care proxy "agent" or "durable power of attorney for health care" is like a mail carrier. He is to carry the patient's messages when the patient cannot deliver them himself. Your mail carrier is not supposed to be writing letters for you. He is just supposed to transmit yours accurately. The only difference is that if the patient did not put his wishes in writing the proxy is authorized to make decisions based on what he was told by the patient or when nothing else is available what is in the best interests of the patient.

In this case, the proxy is a brother who very strongly disagrees with the patient's wishes against transfusion. The patient does not want blood. The proxy must not give consent for the transfusion because that is the wish of the patient. The proxy is not there to wait for a patient to lose capacity and then take over. If this were the case, then no last will and testament would be valid. The last will and testament conveys a person's wishes for their property for when they have died. Death is the ultimate form of loss of decision-making capacity. The executor of the will is to obey the will, not decide what he thinks should have been done.

Never-Competent Person, Best Interests Standard

43. **(d) Ask the guardian what is in the best interests of the patient.**

This patient has never been competent so there is no possibility of trying to determine what he had wanted for himself. There is no family to act in his best interests. You cannot substitute judgment for a person that has never had judgment. This case involves decision making on the least accurate of the decision-making standard, which is to determine what would be in the best interests of the patient. The reason this is the least accurate method of giving or withholding consent is that there is no way to be sure what the patient would have wanted for himself. With a best interests standard we have the difficult problem of determining whether the guardian is basing their decision on what the patient would need, or the guardian's own subjective standard of what they would want for themselves. In this case, the burden of therapy for no chance of cure is worse than the option of simply deferring therapy. If there is a court-appointed guardian, then there is no point of an "expert panel." The question here is not one of what the best medical therapy is, but what is in the best interests of a patient too mentally impaired to make his own decisions.

Pregnant Woman Refusing C-section

44. **(a) Honor her wishes and do not perform the C-section.**

A competent adult has the right to do what she wants with her own body. This is true even if the decision seems foolish or unwise. This is also true even if the patient is pregnant and the fetus is potentially viable. Until the baby is born, a fetus does not have the rights of a "person." An undelivered fetus is judged as a part of the woman's body; hence she has the entire right to choose what will go on. Psychiatry evaluation and a court order are inappropriate because she is fully competent as per the description in this case.

The father does not have the right to decide what to do any more than he has a right to consent to an appendectomy for the mother. The mother's right to refuse a C-section is the same as a mother's right to choose abortion. The father has no say.

Necessity of Informing the Patient of Other Treatment Options

45. **(d) He will win because you did not inform him of the risks and benefits of alternative therapy to surgery.**

    Patients have the right to be fully informed about the risks and benefits of therapy and also about alternative therapies. He cannot make an informed decision if he has not been informed about the alternative to the main course in therapy. The absence of adverse effects does not eliminate the need to tell him the risks of therapy as well as the benefits.

Oral Consent Is Valid

46. **(e) Take consent for the bypass over the phone and have a second person confirm the consent.**

    An oral consent is equal to a written consent if it is valid and provable. The validity of oral consent has nothing to do with the severity of the procedure. If you improperly take consent for a minor procedure you are liable for damages. If you take a proper consent for major surgery it is valid even if it is oral. It is important to have as much documentation of the consent as possible. The second person speaking to the proxy on the phone is a valid way of confirming the consent. A second person should even witness consent in person. There is no limit on what can be consented to by oral consent. It is simply a matter of establishing proof of the consent so no one can deny it later if there is an adverse effect of the procedure.

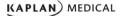

Only a Competent Patient Can Refuse Emergency Lifesaving Procedures

47. **(b) Give the blood.**

   Only a fully conscious patient can refuse a lifesaving blood transfusion. You do not have direct evidence of the patient's wishes for himself. You cannot assume that what the parents are saying is what he would have wanted for himself. If he were awake he may very well say he thinks his parents' religious beliefs are crazy and he wants the blood. He may say he agrees with them. Because you have no clear idea of what the patient wanted for himself, you must give the blood. Consent is implied in an emergency procedure unless there is a contemporary refusal by a conscious patient. You cannot wait for a court hearing. The patient will die in the meantime.

Refusals Made When Competent Are Valid When Capacity Is Lost

48. **(d) You cannot give the blood.**

   The patient has given you a clear advance directive both orally and in writing. You must honor her wishes even if she loses capacity. If this were not true no one would have to honor a person's last will and testament when he or she died. If this were her will and she was designating what she wanted done with her property after death you cannot reassign her property based on what the husband wanted. The most intimate property a person has is her own life and body.

Harm: Intent Not Relevant

49. **(e) The resident and hospital are both liable for harm to the patient.**

Harm exists even if it is unknown to the person acted upon. The intention of the person making the error does not actually matter in terms of assessing both malpractice as well as harm to the patient. In this case, both the resident and hospital are guilty of harm and potentially liable for damages for resulting in an injury to the patient that were avoidable. The nurses and the pharmacist can also be held liable. If a manufacturer sells you a car that is unsafe and you sustain injury they are still liable for damages because it is their responsibility to ensure the safety of the products they sell you. If I own a restaurant and you get food poisoning accidentally from unsafe food or an employee who did not wash his hands, then I am liable. I am not absolved of liability for the harm just because I did not intend harm and am in "good will" toward you. I still harmed you. The same is true of a medication error.

Role of Risk Management

50. **(e) To minimize the legal risk to the hospital from litigation**

Risk management is the term applied to the portion of the hospital administration that evaluates potential legal liability to the institution. The role of risk management is to try to intervene in acute care in a way that primarily protects the hospital from lawsuits. Risk management may lead to better care and communication in the service of reducing the chance that a patient or their family will engage in legal action against the institution.

Informed Consent Protects Against Liability

51. (d) **He loses it because the patient was fully informed about the risks and benefits of both alternatives.**

The key issue in terms of liability for adverse effects to patients is whether the patient was fully informed of the risks of the therapy before the treatment was given. If a major adverse effect or even death occurred, but the patient knew and understood this and still chose to proceed, then there is no liability. The patient was fully informed of what could happen. If a minor adverse effect occurred such as hair loss and the patient was not fully informed that this could occur, then there is wrongdoing. Again, the issue is whether or not the patient gave consent or had the opportunity to make another choice.

The patient's family does not need to be informed. The patient must be informed. IRB approval alone does not shield you from liability. The key issue is whether the patient was given the opportunity to make a free choice.

A man is buying a car. The one in the store he chooses has a cup holder he likes. They deliver a car with a much better engine, but without a cup holder. The dealer is liable because the customer must be given a choice. Maybe he will only buy a car with a cup holder he likes. You cannot say, "This car without the cup holder is a much better car."

It depends on being informed, not on what occurs.

Necessity of Knowing Risks of Deferring Therapy

52. **(e) You lose because you did not inform the patient of the serious consequences of forgoing angioplasty.**

In order for a patient to make an informed consent for a procedure, he must know the risk of not having the procedure done. In this case you did not document that you told the patient that a person with an acute ST segment elevation myocardial infarction who fails to reperfuse with thrombolytics has a markedly increased risk of death without angioplasty. You only informed him of the risks (hematoma, coronary rupture) but not the benefit (decreased mortality) of the procedure. He was not fully informed and therefore you are liable.

In the same way that failing to inform a patient of the risk of harm from doing the procedure is mandatory, you must also inform of the risk of harm when you don't do the procedure.

Duty of Patients to Inform the Staff of Medical Problems

53. **(e) She loses because she did not inform the nurses she was dizzy or lightheaded.**

Malpractice occurs if the physician, hospital, or other staff deviated from the standard of care and the patient sustained harm. It is not a deviation from the standard of care to leave a patient unescorted on the toilet if she does not offer a complaint. There would have been malpractice and liability if the patient had informed the nurses that she was dizzy and in need of assistance and they did not provide it. The patient has a responsibility to inform staff of medical conditions that would have an impact on her care.

KAPLAN MEDICAL

Revealing a Medication Error

54. (c) Apologize and tell the patient that you forgot to reorder the antibiotics, but that he will be all right.

Medical errors are one of the most difficult issues in the ethical management of patients. There are few absolute rules in terms of disclosure and it is one of the most embarrassing issues to deal with. There is very little acceptance of even an honest error on the part of the patient, the physician, or our physician peers. Nevertheless, the ethical direction is clear that you should reveal the error to the patient. The patient has an absolute right to be fully informed about his own care. This means it is his right to know and your duty to inform about any error in care even if there is no demonstrated harm. The patient's right to know is more important than your embarrassment over the error. The greatest obstacle to informing the patient is fear of loss of credibility and the potential loss of confidence of the patient in your competence. The patient may choose to sever the relationship and sometimes to engage in litigation if there is potential harm. You must still tell him the details; it is his right to know.

If you bring your car for repair and the mechanic makes a mistake in the repair, you are entitled to know. The car is your property and no one has a right to mismanage your property without your knowledge. The most personal form of property is your own body.

Disagreements Between Residents and Attendings

55. (e) Bring the disagreement to the chief of service.

Your first duty is to the patient; however, you cannot damage the physician/patient relationship between the private attending and the patient. You cannot just change therapy on someone's patient without his knowledge. It would be inappropriate to go outside your local hierarchy without first appealing privately to the chief of service. The chief of service has the authority in an institution to intervene in quality of care issues.

Absolute Right of Patients to View Their Own Records

56. **(d) She has the right to her own records even without giving a reason.**

The patient does not have to provide a reason for why she wants a copy of her records. The reasons for desiring the record are not pertinent. The medical record cannot be withheld from the patient for any reason including nonpayment of bills. The patient's health-care information cannot be held like a hostage for ransom. This right is so strong, that it is actually the physician, hospital, and insurance provider who must seek the patient's approval in order for them to get a copy of the patient's records. You, as a physician, require written permission from the patient in order for you to get a copy of the records from another institution.

Ownership of Medical Records

57. **(c) The information is the property of the patient and the physical paper or electronic record is the property of the health-care provider.**

The health-care provider can provide copies of the medical record to the patient or other health-care providers, but the physical record is the property of the physician, clinic, or hospital. Hence, the original record always remains with the provider of care. The information in the record is the property of the patient and that is why the patient is entitled to access of the chart.

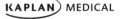

Changing Inaccuracies in the Record

58. (e) **Write a new note with the current date and time.**

The two methods of correcting errors in documentation are to place a single line through the original error, write in the new information, and add your initials or to place an entirely new note with the current date and time. Use the first method if you find the error immediately and the timing is the same. The reason not to remove, erase, or use correction fluid on the error is to maintain credibility. If you alter the note in an unacceptable way, then the thought process—including the mistake—cannot be followed. You must never backdate/postdate a note. You cannot rewrite history by trying to make it look like a note written today was really written yesterday. Always use the current date and time for what you write in the chart.

Informed Consent Mandatory for Suturing

59. (c) **Wait for the consent of at least one parent.**

This is not an emergency procedure and can wait for consent of a parent. Procedures that are emergencies do not need any informed consent from a parent in order to begin the treatment. We do not want a child's health to suffer just because no one is present to give consent at that moment an emergency occured. Neighbors cannot give consent. Only parents or legal guardians can give consent for procedures for minors; however you do not need both parents to sign consent. You would only seek a court-appointed guardian if there were no identifiable parents. This patient cannot give consent because he is a minor, which in most states is defined as being under age 18. By definition, minors are considered incompetent except on areas of oral contraceptives, STDs, prenatal care, and rehabilitation or detoxification for substance abuse.

STD in a Minor

60. **(a) Ceftriaxone/azithromycin now in a single dose.**

Parental consent is not required to treat a minor for illnesses such as sexually trans-mitted diseases (STDs), prenatal care, contraception, HIV, or substance abuse. A minor is defined as a person under the age of 18. Parental consent is required for all other forms of treatment other than these with the exception of emergency treat-ment. In this case, although cervicitis is not an emergency, she can receive treatment without even trying to notify the parents. We want to lower the barriers to the care of these diseases. In other words, we prevent more STDs and unwanted pregnancies by granting a minor full access to this form of care. The requirement for parental con-sent makes the minor less likely to come in for care. Less STD treatment means more transmission. Less contraceptive management means more unwanted pregnancies. There is no consensus nationally on parental notification for abortion. Some states require it and some don't.

Urgent Blood Transfusion in the Child of a Jehovah's Witness

61. **(c) Give blood to the child but not to the father.**

Any competent adult may refuse therapy of any kind, including the lifesaving ones. The same is not true for a minor. Minors cannot refuse urgent lifesaving therapy. That is why the father may refuse for himself, but not for the child. This question does not address whether the child wants the blood or not. The child's wishes in a matter of urgent, lifesaving therapy are not relevant to the proper ethical treatment of the child. A 12-year-old child, by definition, is treated as you would an incompetent adult. That is, you are happy if they are agreeable, but you will still do what you think is right anyway. In a legal sense, a minor child is like your dog. You are happy if he doesn't bark during the treatment, but you will not change your method of treatment based on his opinion. You do not need a court order in this case because the direction is clear and well worked out. You save the life of the child; don't wait.

KAPLAN) MEDICAL

There is no need for a psychiatric evaluation because the father was clearly competent and it doesn't matter what the child says. Intravenous iron will not work fast enough. The cases must be clear and unequivocal. Occasionally, a 17-year-old child with leukemia that will likely be fatal anyway is allowed to refuse a transfusion or chemotherapy. This sort of case is far, far different. A 17-year-old is close to a legal adult, the disease is not sudden, and the treatment will likely not change outcome.

The bottom line is that parents cannot refuse lifesaving therapy for a child.

Prenatal Care in a Minor

62.   (a) **"I will give you the care you need and keep it confidential."**

Prenatal care is one of the exceptions to the general rule of parental notification and consent for the treatment of minors. You do not have to inform either the parents of the patient or the father of the baby. This confidentiality also extends to protecting the patient even if the parents were to ask. The patient has a right to privacy for her prenatal care.

Emergency Treatment of a Minor

63.   (d) **Perform the appendectomy.**

The patient described in this case has acute appendicitis and needs an urgent procedure. An appendectomy must be performed as soon as possible in acute appendicitis. You cannot allow harm to the patient because you are momentarily unable to contact the parents. Intravenous antibiotics alone are insufficient to treat acute appendicitis. Again, you cannot harm the child because the parents are not able to be located at this moment. Only a parent or legal guardian can consent to a procedure on a patient. Neighbors, aunt and uncles, grandparents, and babysitters cannot give consent for a child that is not their own. Minor children cannot consent to an appendectomy.

Emancipated Minor

64. (d) "I will give you the isotretinoin as requested."

This patient, although a minor, is a special exemption known as an "emancipated minor." This category applies to persons who are under the age of 18 but who are independent of their parents. An emancipated minor is one who is either self-supporting, married, in the military, or who has children that they are supporting through their own independent means such as their own job. A large portion of the definition of an emancipated minor has to do with the patient being self-supporting and living independently. There is no definite age cutoff for when someone may be considered an emancipated minor. The age varies by state but is usually at either age 15 or 16. An emancipated minor is capable of consenting to any medical procedure. All minors can consent to prenatal, contraception, HIV, STD, and substance abuse care. An emancipated minor is one that can consent to any form of care or procedure as if he or she was an adult.

65. (a) Provide the pain medications as appropriate but not the means to end his life.

Physician-assisted suicide is always considered unacceptable. The patient is not acutely depressed so antidepressants are unnecessary. This form of reasoning does not need an inpatient psychiatric evaluation. Try never to refer patients on board questions for anything. There is no "specialist" that can certify a patient as a good candidate for assisted suicide. There is an ethical imperative for the physician to preserve life. Consequently there are no acceptable circumstances in which a patient can act as an assistant in suicide. There is significant concern that putting the power to end life in the hands of the physician is an uncontrollable power that would easily be subject to abuse and indiscriminant use. In addition, there may be many depressed persons in need of treatment for depression who would otherwise simply choose suicide on demand. Remember that the boards are not testing your personal opinions about what you think ought to be acceptable. They are testing the best consensus of the law and practice guidelines.

KAPLAN MEDICAL

You may personally agree with physician-assisted suicide or disagree that first trimester abortions are acceptable. Just do not choose these as the answers to the test questions. Forty-nine or 50 states have laws that make physician-assisted suicide illegal. The experiment in the state of Oregon where physician-assisted suicide is legal does not hold true for any other place in the United States. Hence, on a national examination, you must go with what would be true in the majority of cases. In addition, despite whatever laws there are currently, all physician professional groups consider assisted suicide unethical.

Lethal Injection Always Unacceptable

66. **(e) You tell him that under no circumstances can you participate in euthanasia.**

Under no circumstances is it ethical for a physician to participate in euthanasia. The difference between euthanasia and physician-assisted suicide is that euthanasia is a means of death administered to the patient by another. Physicians are not ethically permitted to destroy life. This is true even if there is a law authorizing it. The higher ethical duty of the physician to preserve life supersedes state law. Euthanasia is unacceptable even if a competent patient requests it. Physician-assisted suicide is different from euthanasia in that the physician provides the patient with the means to end their own lives. In physician-assisted suicide, the patient administers the means of ending their life. In euthanasia, the physician administers the means of death. Both of these are unacceptable. This is markedly different from giving pain medications or other therapy that inadvertently ends the patient's life. If the only way to control a person's pain and suffering completely is to give medications that inadvertently or unintentionally shorten the patient's life, this is acceptable. This is sometimes referred to as terminal sedation. The primary issue is one of intent. In euthanasia, the primary intent is to end life. In terminal sedation, the primary intent is to relieve suffering.

Substance-Abusing Resident

67. **(e) Report him to the chairperson or program director of his department.**

The reporting of a potentially impaired physician is an ethical duty that cannot be bypassed. Although you have an absolute duty to protect the patients under his care, you should first go to the person in the table of organization to whom the resident reports. Telling your dean of students is inappropriate because the dean of students does not supervise the resident. Telling the dean of students would be appropriate if the impaired person was another student. For physicians-in-training the first stop is their program director or department chair. For attending physicians it can be the department chair or the medical director of the hospital. For attending physicians not reporting or working for local authorities, make the report at the higher level of the state licensing board or the mechanisms in place for impaired physicians. It is fruitless to go straight to the impaired person. It is like reporting child abuse. If the person who is impaired admits it to you, you must still report centrally to make sure of the follow-up and resolution. If they deny the problem you must still do the same.

If you notice the impairment and do not report it, then you become liable for any harm that might happen to a patient.

Dementia in Attending

68. **(d) Report him to the state licensing board.**

Reports of physician impairment should go first to the local supervisory personnel. If this is either unsuccessful or not applicable then report it to a higher level such as a state licensing board. Telling your own division head is inappropriate because that person supervises you, not the potentially impaired physician.

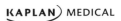

Behavior Abnormalities Not Affecting Patient Care

69. **(d) Do nothing.**

Your responsibility for reporting physician impairment rests only with reporting abnormalities that may affect patient care. If there are no abnormalities in her ability to make medical decisions and supervise junior house officers then to report details of a physician's personal life would only be potential slander. Loss of reputation is a serious issue for a physician. Other physicians and patients will not want to use a physician whom they think is of low moral character even if her medical care is fine. You do not have to agree with, condone, or approve of the behavior you witness. However, there has to be evidence of medical impropriety in order for it to be worthy of being reported. The Committee on Physician Impairment helps physicians with substance problem. This is before they drive or manage patients while intoxicated. If a physician is impaired and takes care of patients while intoxicated, then the physician should be reported to the local chief of service or Department of Health.

Right Not to Accept Patients

70. **(a) It is both legal and ethical.**

There is no legal or ethical mandate to care for any patient who comes to see you. The physician/patient relationship must be entered into voluntarily on both parts. Hence, if the physician's practice is full, there is no obligation to accept new patients. It would be unethical if the physician were to accept some patients based on arbitrary personal preferences and reject others for the same reason, although this is not illegal. For example, it would be unethical to accept or reject patients simply on the basis of race, gender, or religion unless it had to do with a specific area of expertise such as being a gynecologist rejecting male patients. Although it is courteous to make a referral to another physician there is no obligation to arrange for care from another physician. This is entirely different from a case in which a patient was already under the care of a physician. In this case, a physician must arrange for appropriate transfer to another physician's care as he ends the relationship. Once having accepted responsibility for a patient there is far less freedom on the part of the physician to break that relationship. To cease from providing care to an ill patient without appropriate transfer of care is both an unethical and illegal action characterized as patient abandonment.

Duty to the Patient, Gag Orders Not Valid, HMO

71. (a) **Fully inform the patient about the risks and benefits of bone marrow transplantation.**

Your primary duty is always to the patient. One of the unique elements of the physician/patient relationship is that its ethical boundaries transcend ordinary rules of the workplace and institutional rules. As such, you cannot withhold information from a patient if that information may lead to benefit for the patient. In order to make an "informed consent," the patient must be fully informed. The patient cannot be fully informed if he has not heard of the options. It is not appropriate for you to back away from educating your patient by transferring care unless it is for an area outside your expertise. There is no need to encourage litigation under any circumstances.

It is not ethical to tell a patient about a potential therapy only if he asks about it. It is our duty to inform him. "Gag orders" preventing the education of patients about treatment options are always wrong. The patients cannot have autonomy over the choice of treatment of their body if they are not aware of the options. Beneficence to the patient always outweighs institutional directives.

Physicial Refusing to Treat HIV Patients for a Procedure

72. **(e)** **Refer the patient to another cardiothoracic surgeon.**

The patient has a very clear need for coronary bypass surgery with three-vessel disease and left ventricular function. The bottom-line point to this question is about what you do for patients who need a particular procedure when the physician is refusing to do the right thing. Answers b, c, and d involve switching the patient to another form of therapy, which is inadequate, compared with surgery. This is unacceptable. You cannot force the surgeon to operate against his will. Although it is unethical for a physician to refuse care on the basis of race, gender, ethnic origin, and diseases such as HIV, you cannot legally force a physician to take care of someone they do not want to. The physician/patient relationship that must be entered into voluntarily on both parts; hence, it is unethical to refuse to treat a patient solely based on your dislike or discomfort with HIV-positive persons, but it is not illegal. The chief of service may have the power to remove or suspend hospital privileges and to fire someone for unethical behavior, but the chief of service does not have the ability to force a physician to perform a procedure. When a patient needs a procedure that your consultant will not do, then the right action is to find the patient a doctor who will do the right thing. Although this case was framed in terms of HIV, the answer of referring to another physician would be the same no matter what reason the physician had for refusing to do the procedure.

Sexual Relations between Physician and Patient

73. **(d)** **"I cannot date you and be your doctor—maybe in the future we can date, after you get another doctor."**

Sexual relations between a physician and a current patient are never ethically acceptable. At the very least, the physician/patient relationship must stop. The patient must transfer her care to another physician. This is to avoid an abuse of power in the relationship and to keep clear boundaries. Relationships between a psychiatrist and a patient are generally never acceptable even after the physician/patient relationship has stopped. It does not matter who initiates the relationship. There is no ethics board in place to act as a dating service for physicians.

74   **(c) Herpes simplex**

The primary purpose of reporting diseases to the Department of Health is to be able to interrupt a cycle of transmission. In addition, we wish to know the epidemiology of diseases in order to assess resource allocation and the success of intervention programs. Finally, for infectious diseases we report sensitivity patterns in order to guide appropriate empiric therapy in the future. For instance, we track the sensitivity of gonorrhea resistance to quinolones in order to assess whether we can continue to use quinolones empirically to treat patients into the future. We report salmonella so that we can identify and eliminate the source of the infection such as a restaurant closed or contaminated food discarded. We report tuberculosis so that the contacts can be PPD skin-tested and the source patient isolated until noninfectious. Measles notification is important so that we can assess who needs vaccines in order to prevent further spread. Herpes does not need any of these interventions. Herpes spreads only through intimate contact. It cannot spread through contaminated food and water like salmonella. Herpes cannot be effectively eradicated from the entire body. In between outbreaks, herpes is dormant in the body and the outbreaks only shorten with abortive therapy such as acyclovir. People often harbor asymptomatic gonorrhea, which can be detected and eradicated. There is no isolation for herpes and there is no effective vaccine.

Tuberculosis Isolation and Incarceration

75.   **(d) Remove the patient from his job as a bus driver and incarcerate him in a hospital to take medications.**

The patient's right to privacy and autonomy ends when the public's right to safety is at risk. The patient does not have the right to be at-large with persistently positive sputum stains for acid-fast bacilli. You do not have the right to force feed the medications through a nasogastric tube, but you do have the right to remove the patient from his job and put him in a hospital where he cannot infect others until his sputum is free of acid-fast bacilli. This is not just because he has a job as a bus driver, which has a lot of contact with the public. TB incarceration is not the same as being arrested. It is part of the Department of Health, not the criminal justice system. You go to a hospital where the only way to get out is to take the medications and have clean sputum. You do not go to a jail.

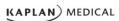

Partner Notification for Syphilis

76. **(d) The Department of Health will send a letter or call the contacts and let them know they have a serious health issue. They will test and treat the partners but will not reveal his name.**

The need to keep the population free from disease limits the patient's right to privacy. You have a duty to the other contacts he may have infected. However, in order to respect the patients' privacy, the Department of Health has never revealed the name of the source patient, no matter how much they are asked. They make the original notification by phone or mail but only reveal the specific disease in person. If the patient won't reveal the names of his contacts, you have no means to force him to do so. You cannot incarcerate or arrest a patient because he will not reveal the names of his contacts.

Physician Objecting to Performing Abortions

77. **(e) Refer the patient for the abortion.**

Patients have the legal right to safe and effective abortions. This right is universal within the first trimester and no further evaluation or waiting period is required. The right to abortion after the first trimester (12 weeks) is less clear, and extenuating circumstances such as a risk to the life of the mother from the pregnancy or whether the conception is a product of sexual assault are also considered. The criteria for ready access to abortion becomes less clear after the first trimester as the fetus progresses in its development toward becoming a viable infant.

Although you may object to abortion, the patient still has a legal right to obtain one. You are not under an obligation to perform the abortion yourself. Your objection can cover your refusal to do the procedure personally but you do not have the right to refuse to refer her to the care she needs as your patient. Although a physician has the right to refuse to enter into the physician/patient relationship before it has begun, once you have entered into the relationship you are obligated to provide the care the patient needs. Hence, you cannot just terminate the physician/patient relationship at the moment the patient needs a form of care you disagree with. You cannot ask for a four-week waiting period especially when the patient presents at eight weeks of pregnancy and this wait will bring her past the first trimester.

If the patient has clear decision-making capacity, there is no need to obtain a psychological evaluation.

Parental Notification for Abortion

78. **(e) Strongly encourage her to discuss the issue with her parents.**

Although competent adults have an unfettered legal right to abortion within the first trimester, this right is not universal for a minor. A minor is generally defined as a person below the age of 18. The necessity of parental consent or at least notification is a mixed issue across states nationally. Some states require parental notification and some states do not. Hence, as a board examination, which is given nationally, there is no single clear answer. Unlike the bar examination for lawyers, physicians take virtually no state-specific examination. When you pass USMLE or the Board of Internal Medicine, it is valid in every state.

The only thing that is always clear is that we should strongly encourage the patient herself to have the discussion with her parents. Many of the boards will want an answer indicating discussion before action so you will be trained into trying to build consensus. Even if you are within your rights to walk up to a brain-dead patient and remove the ventilator without consent of the family, the boards will always want you to answer "discuss with the family" first if that is one of the options.

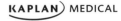

KAPLAN) MEDICAL

Sterilization—Husband Disagrees

79. (a) Refer for the tubal ligation as requested by the wife.

Although it is preferable to have consensus, there is absolutely no spousal consent required for sterilization procedures of either partner. The fallopian tubes are located within the body of the woman; hence it is a matter of her right to autonomy over her own body that she has the right to the sterilization procedure if that is what she desires. The number of children that a patient has bears no impact on the acceptability of the sterilization procedure. If this were true, it would be equivalent to legally mandating that every woman must reproduce. In other words, "We will tie your tubes, only as long as you have put them to good use. First fulfill your biological potential, and then we will sterilize you." This is unacceptable reasoning. A woman has a right to choose what to do with her own body. If a man buys a new car but chooses never to drive it, that is his right. If he chooses to throw out the car, that is his right. You cannot mandate that he drive the car because the car is new. You cannot tell him he must keep the car because "you might change your mind later, and want to go for a drive."

As long as there is no evidence of psychiatric disturbance or incapacity to understand her medical issues, a psychological evaluation is not necessary.

Paternal Consent for Abortion Not Necessary

80. (e) You say you have an absolute duty to the mother to honor her wishes no matter what his personal feelings are.

A woman has a right to choose what to do with her own body. Undelivered babies or fetuses do not have legal standing as an independent person to bring a suit to prevent its termination. Until the moment of delivery, the embryo is considered an extension of the woman's body. She does not need consent from the father of the child or any member of the family. Her ability to consent to the termination is equal to her consent for a breast biopsy or a leg amputation.

Although a fetus may genetically contain half the genetic elements of both parents, it is the female that must go through the delivery. Hence, the woman has a "right of ownership" over any undelivered child because it inhabits her body.

Third Trimester Abortion

81. **(d) Legally you can only do it if her life is at risk.**

Abortion during the third trimester is the most controversial area of reproductive rights. There is no automatic right to abortion on demand past the first trimester. During the third trimester, the fetus is potentially viable. A fetus at 28 weeks of gestational age (six months) can potentially survive intact with a delivery although it would have a greater risk of complications secondary to prematurity. The Supreme Court has consistently left exceptions for the possibility of abortion in later stages of pregnancy if the life of the mother is at risk. You cannot ethically freely abort a potentially viable fetus unless there is a very significant extenuating circumstance such as risk to the mother or a fetus so developmentally abnormal that fetal demise is certain.

As for a court order, the court cannot order a physician to perform a task that is ethically or professionally unacceptable. For example, if a law passed tomorrow making it legal to perform euthanasia on a person with Down syndrome, it would still be unethical to do so even with a court order. This is similar to the ethical unacceptability of a physician participating in an execution. The condemned is under a court order to die and it is legal. However, it is unethical for a physician to participate, as a physician, in an execution.

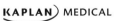

Victim Objects to Reporting

82. (b) **You will report the injury only with his consent.**

The rules on the reporting of domestic violence are much less strict than those on reporting child abuse are. This is because a competent adult has the voluntary choice of reporting the injury themselves in the vast majority of cases. In addition, you cannot violate the patient's right to autonomy by specifically doing something that has expressively been refused. For children there is mandatory reporting because children do not have the ability to defend themselves. Minors, by definition, are deemed incompetent except for a few exceptions like sexually transmitted diseases (STDs). Children are not, therefore, considered to have autonomy that can be violated.

This patient is being physically abused. As an adult patient with the capacity to understand his medical problems, he has the right to refuse care and protection from reporting the injury if that is what he wants.

Attempted Suicide—Need for Emergency Procedure

83. (b) **Perform the surgery.**

This patient's injury is, in a sense, the same as a purposeful drug overdose, jumping off a bridge, or trying to shoot himself. In this case, the car is a large gun. Although an adult patient with the capacity to understand his medical care can refuse treatment, this is not the same as allowing patients to kill themselves. People actively trying to kill themselves are, by definition, not considered competent. The right to autonomy ends just short of condoning active suicide. It is assumed, in this case, that the suicide attempt was performed while under the intolerable emotional burden of recently having found he had cancer. An assumption is made that when acute life stressors lead a patient to attempt suicide that they are temporarily incompetent and psychotherapy or psychopharmacology may help him. If you review the question you will see that the case never stated that the cancer was incurable, progressive, or even fatal.

You cannot let a patient kill himself while under acute psychological distress such as depression. You cannot wait for a court order for emergency surgery in a hemorrhaging patient. The family's consent is not necessary. It is nice to have, but does not alter the reasoning stated above. If I was trying to commit suicide, it would not matter if my family comes by and says, "It's okay, let him die." You still have to intervene to prevent the active suicide.

Not Ethical to Participate in Physical Torture

84. (e) **You cannot participate in the purposeful torture of a prisoner.**

Physicians are never ethically allowed to participate in the torture of anyone. This is true even if there is a court order directing you to do so. It would not be ethical to assault someone or murder someone even if there is a court order. The physician's duty to the patient transcends duty to ordinary institutional structure. This is true even if the prisoner has been convicted of the crime. We cannot have our duty to patients flexible based on whether they have been accused, arrested, charged, on trial, or convicted. It is always unethical to participate in the purposeful injury whether physical or psychological of a prisoner. There is no release you can obtain from a superior or an institution that makes unethical behavior ethical. The physician cannot later justify participation in torture under the rubric, "I was only following orders."

Duty to Report Injury to Prisoners

85. (a) **Report the injuries as signs of possible torture.**

You have a duty to protect the welfare of all patients under your care. This includes prisoners. Failing to report the injury makes you an accomplice or in some sense participatory to the injury because you did nothing to prevent the next injury. This duty transcends your presence either in or out of the military. It would be the same as finding evidence of child abuse. You are a mandated reporter. You are liable if you fail to report an injury to a child that you suspect of being abuse. If there is a subsequent injury to the child, those who fail to report the first injury are liable for helping to cause the subsequent injury by failing to report the first. The same is true for evidence of torture to prisoners. You have an ethical duty to report even if the injury turns out not to have been secondary to torture.

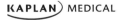

Hence, in terms of torture and child abuse, the physician's ethical duty is to detect and report possible episodes. There is no obligation to only report episodes that are always proven to be episodes of abuse or torture.

Futile Treatment

86.   (e) Recommend that dialysis not be performed

You are not required to administer any form of therapy that you feel would be futile. You do not have to perform the dialysis if it will not lead to any significant benefit for the patient. This is true even if the family is requesting that you perform the dialysis. Although, in practice, it is extremely difficult not to honor a family's wishes to perform any therapy, there is no legal or ethical requirement to do so. In this case, besides the persistent vegetative state, there is multiorgan failure associated with essentially no chance of survival. Hence, dialysis would not be prolonging this patient's life; it would only be prolonging the dying process. In this case, doing dialysis would ethically be the same as the family requesting kidney transplantation.

Adult with Capacity Requesting Withdrawal of Ventilator

87.   (a) Remove the ventilator as she requests.

Any adult patient with the capacity to understand her medical problems has the right to do what she wishes with her own body. Although there may be an emotional distinction on the part of the caregivers and family between withholding of care and withdrawal of care, there is no ethical or legal distinction. This patient understands she will die and it is her legal right to have the ventilator removed if she wishes. A court order is not necessary because this type of case has been legally worked out in the past in other cases. The consent of the family and the proxy are not necessary because the patient is alert and able to communicate her own wishes. The health-care proxy only becomes responsible for decision making when the patient loses the capacity to speak for herself. You should not even consult the proxy and the family when the patient is alert unless it is at the request of the patient. Sedation is inappropriate. We cannot just sedate people when we do not like their decisions. You do not have the right to force any form of therapy on a competent patient. This would be different only if the person were acutely suicidal.

Adult with Capacity Refusing Lifesaving Chemotherapy

88. (d) **Honor the patient's wishes.**

The patient is an adult who has the capacity to understand the risks and benefits of therapy. Consequently she has the right to refuse or accept therapy or any part of the therapy that she sees fit. Psychiatric evaluation would only be necessary if there were evidence of depression and possible suicidal ideation. Psychiatry evaluation is also useful sometimes if the patient's capacity to understand her medical condition is unclear. If the patient clearly understands her issues or is clearly unable to understand then a psychiatric evaluation is unnecessary. The court has no standing to appoint a guardian to overrule an adult with the capacity to understand her issues. Radiotherapy is not adequate therapy for stage III lymphoma. In addition, you cannot substitute another therapy without the patient's consent. Risk management is an institutional agent whose role is to minimize the risk of litigation for the institution. They would not be necessary here as long as you have adequately documented the patient's mental capacity and the refusal of therapy.

Depressed Patient Refusing Therapy

89. (a) **Psychiatric evaluation.**

This patient is severely depressed with vegetative signs of depression such as weight change, anhedonia, and sleep disturbance. It is important to evaluate and treat depression, which may be a temporary condition, prior to withholding therapy without which the patient will likely die. In addition, the shortness of breath may indicate hypoxia, which may be interfering with the patient's capacity to understand their medical condition. You do not want to sedate a patient who needs to speak to a psychiatrist. In addition, simply sedating a patient who is refusing therapy may be construed as simply making him unable to refuse therapy. The family's opinion does not change the primary duty to the patient to assure that the reason for the refusal of potentially lifesaving therapy is not simply untreated depression. Ethics committee evaluation is most useful when a patient does not have the capacity to understand his medical condition and the family members are in disagreement. A DNR order does not absolve you of the need to treat the patient's other conditions.

KAPLAN) MEDICAL

Refusal of Artificial Nutrition; Disagreement with the Proxy

90. **(d) Do not place any form of tube for artificial nutrition or hydration.**

Your primary duty is to the patient who specifically told you not to place any form of tube for artificial nutrition. Although the proxy has the ability to overrule anyone in the family in terms of decision making, she cannot overrule the patient. Although the paper documentation did not specifically mention J-tube, the patient gave you a clear oral advance directive and that is the absolute rule. You must stick by it no matter what a court or the ethics committee may say. Although it is your right to refuse to accept a patient, you cannot ethically transfer the care of a patient to someone who will go against the patient's wishes just because you feel uncomfortable. Oral advance directives are harder to prove but they are still valid. This is true even when the patient loses the capacity to make decisions. If we did not honor a patient's wishes after losing competence, no one would be able to make a last will and testament. A person's will is, in essence, a proxy directing the financial and property wishes of the patient. Death is the ultimate way of losing capacity to make decisions. A person's advance directive is a form of will directing what he wishes done with the most personal property a patient can have: his own life and body.

Proxy as Ultimate Decision Maker

91. **(a) Honor the proxy and do not intubate.**

The health-care proxy is the ultimate decision maker in all matters of health care. When the patient loses capacity to make decisions. The proxy is the designee by the patient to determine and implement the patient's wishes in the event that a patient becomes unable to make decisions. It does not matter if every single person in the universe wants a particular therapy if there is a proxy that accurately knows the wishes of the patient. The proxy overrules the mother every time because the proxy is the person designated by the patient to make judgments for the patient's care. The proxy is like the executor of a will. Although a consensus agreement with the family is not necessary sometimes the questions contain an answer choice that says "encourage discussions" amongst the family and proxy or "seek agreement." When that answer is present it is usually the right choice. It is always better to seek consensus and agreement through discussion. An ethics committee evaluation is not necessary if either there is a proxy who knows the definite wishes of the patient or, when there is no proxy, when there is agreement amongst the family. Neurology consultation is not necessary for the same reason.

It is like voting. If you have a letter from a person with their proxy ballot for an election, it does not matter what other people think; you cast the vote the patient wanted. Not the vote that his mother thinks is best for him. When a patient documents clear wishes, the proxy is like a mail carrier delivering the record of the patient's plan for himself.

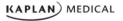

No Proxy, Disagreement amongst Family

92.   (a) **Encourage discussion amongst the family.**

When there is no clear evidence of a patient's wishes for himself, we must seek the best evidence we can find of what judgment the patient would make for himself were he awake and communicative. In practice this is not a problem as long as the family members all agree. In addition, when there is disagreement, particularly when the family members are considered to have equal "weight" then we must first try to seek consensus by encouraging discussion. Only if this is not fruitful should an outside third party such as the courts be sought. All necessary therapy should continue while the evidence of the patient's wishes is collected.

No Proxy, Disagreement amongst Family, No Consensus

93.   (e) **Pursue an ethics committee evaluation.**

When there is no clear evidence of the patient's wishes, then you must seek the best "substituted judgment." The physician must seek out what the patient would have wished for herself and you "substitute" the judgment of the caregivers or family for what the patient would have wanted for herself had she been awake. When a reachable consensus by discussion is not possible then an evaluation by the ethics committee is appropriate to seek consensus. This is the weakest form of decision making because it carries the least precision. If a clear agreement still is unreachable then referral to the courts may be necessary to achieve clarity and objectively weigh the evidence that the different family members bring forth. This is what happened in the Terry Schiavo case in which the patient's husband was judged by the courts as bringing the best evidence that he and others had the most accurate knowledge of what the patient wanted for herself.

If there is no family available then the ethics committee and physicians would make decisions based on the judgment of what would be in the best interests of the patient.

Terminal Sedation, Palliative Care, "Double-Effect"

94. (b) It is acceptable as long as the patient understands the risks.

Your primary duty to a patient with a terminal condition and intractable pain is to relieve suffering. It is unacceptable and unethical to leave him to suffer. As long as he understands that the pain medications may have the "double-effect" of both relieving his pain and possible shortening his life and he agrees then it is acceptable. It is the same as performing a risky surgical procedure in which the patient consents to a lifesaving surgery knowing there is a risk of possible death. This is the same as cardiac bypass grafting in which the surgery will prolong life if successful, but has a risk of death from the procedure. This is the same as a bone marrow transplantation in which the patient has a very significant risk of death, but must do it in order to prevent death from leukemia. A DNR order alone is not a way of avoiding risk. Physician-assisted suicide is illegal in virtualy all jurisdictions. You cannot purposely end the patient's life.

The primary issue is the intent of the physician in giving the pain medications. If the primary aim is to relieve suffering and there is an inadvertent shortening of life as an adverse effect, then it is acceptable. If the primary intent is to end his life with the medications then it is unacceptable.

The direct statement of the U.S. Supreme Court is "the state permits physicians to administer medication to patients in terminal conditions where the primary intent is to relieve pain, even when the medication is so powerful as to hasten death and the patient chooses to receive it with that understanding."

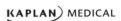

Validity of the Living Will

95. **(c) Remove the tube and the ventilator.**

All adults of sound mind have the right to do what they want with their own body. The patient has left a clear advance directive of what she wanted clearly stating she does not want ventilator management if there is no hope of recovery. It does not matter what the risk manager, the rest of the family, or even the husband wants. All that matters is what the patient wanted. To treat a patient for anything without her consent is legally equivalent to assault and battery. In this case, if you leave the ventilator in place you are "mugging" the patient. This case is extremely clear because the advance directive is in writing and specifies the precise medical intervention that is being refused by name. A court order is unnecessary because the courts do not have the authority to treat a patient against her will.

The vast majority of states have actual statutes saying that a living will is a valid form of advance directive that absolutely must be honored. All 50 states have laws declaring the validity of advance directives. In the three states that do not have specific living will statues, there is case law and legal precedent showing that the living will must be honored. It is clearer if we take the word "living" out of the reasoning and view the patient's body as a house in which the husband brings in a will directing what she wants done with her house. If the document is valid then you must honor it no matter what the rest of the family or the courts say.

No Capacity, No Proxy, No Limitation on What Can Be Withdrawn by Family in Consensus

96. **(e) Nothing**

There is no limitation on what family can withdraw that is united in agreeing on the wishes of the patient. The difficulties arise when the family splits in their opinion as to what the patient wanted. The best form of advance directive is a proxy with an agent that has the patient's wishes for herself written out and described by specific procedure. In other words, instead of saying "no heroic measures" the proxy says "no mechanical ventilation, no nasogastric tube placement, and no artificial nutrition." This is the patient speaking for herself. It is clear and precise. There are no limits on what can be withdrawn or withheld. When this is not present, then the family or friends must describe what the patient would have wanted for herself had she been able to speak. In this case the family acts as a substitute for the judgment of the patient themselves. Substituted judgment is not as good as a proxy because there is no clear documentation. The family is stating what they believe are the patient's wishes for themselves. This is the case in this question. Because they are in agreement, there is no problem. They can do anything including pulling out the endotracheal tube and stopping nasogastric tube feeding.

The pivotal point is that the family is conveying what they understand the patient would wish for herself, not what they think is right for the patient. The last form of decision making for a patient without decision-making capacity and without a proxy is people making a judgment of what they think is in the best interests of the patient. This form of decision making of the "best interest" standard is when there is no documentation of the patient's wishes (living will), and no proxy.

The order of directives arranged from strongest to weakest is:

1. Adult with capacity—No limit on what can be withdrawn/withheld

2. No capacity, but with proxy that states in writing the patient's wishes—No limitation

3. No capacity, no proxy, but written wishes from the patient—No limitation

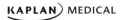

4. No capacity, no proxy, no written wishes, but family united in knowing the patient's wishes (essentially a verbal advance directive)—No limitation

When there is no proxy and no living will and the family is not in agreement, then an arbitration process should occur starting with an institutional ethics committee and sometimes ending in the courts.

Adult with Capacity Wants to Stop Artificial Nutrition

97. (a) **"I will get that tube out right away, sir."**

An adult patient with the capacity to understand his medical problems has the right to stop any form of therapy he wants to. This patient gives the reason that he is uncomfortable, however, the patient does not have to give you any reason. He can just say, "I do not want it," and you must stop. There is no evidence of psychosis or depression described in the case so there is no reason to doubt the decision-making capacity of the patient.

When the patient has the capacity to understand, the wishes of the family, the courts, or the proxy are not relevant to what you have to comply with in terms of the patient's care.

There is a big difference between not complying with a patient's wishes for himself and not agreeing with the decision. You do not have to agree with a competent person's wishes for himself, but you do have to comply with them.

Removing tube feeding in a person who needs the nutrition has a different emotional feeling for many caregivers because it seems like denying basic comfort. Nevertheless, there is no legal or ethical distinction. Tube feedings are a medical intervention that can stop like any other at the discretion of the patient. You cannot force-feed a patient against their will.

Competent Adult Wants to Stop Dialysis

98. (f) "Although I disagree with your decision, I will stop the dialysis."

An adult with the capacity to understand the effects of his decisions can stop any form of therapy even if it will lead to his death. Stopping dialysis is not a form of physician-assisted suicide or euthanasia. Euthanasia means giving a medication that will kill the patient. The primary difference is one of intent. Passive dying from stopping a medical treatment is entirely at the discretion of the patient provided that the person is not acutely depressed and suicidal. By definition, a suicidal patient is deemed not to be competent. This case specifically states that the patient is not depressed.

Although there may be an emotional difference between stopping therapy and ever starting in the first place, there is no legal difference. There is no ethical or legal difference between withholding and withdrawing a treatment. All that matters is that you are adhering to a competent adult's clear wishes for his own care.

If I am painting your house blue and halfway through the job you insist that I paint the house red, I must comply with your wishes. I can't tell you, "Sorry, once I start to paint, I don't stop until the job is done. Your wishes are less important than mine." It is your house. You can do what you want with it.

Adult without Capacity and a Vague Living Will

99. (a) Continue both for now.

The major difficulty with the living will is that it is often not clear and specific in terms of what it means. The phrase "no heroic measures" is not sufficiently clear as an advance directive to stop a ventilator that the person's life is dependent upon. You also do not know if the patient's wishes have changed since the last visit. As far as you know, the patient's family may appear any minute and say the patient wants to be on a ventilator as long as it is not permanent. They may say "no heroic measures" meant dialysis and organ transplantation in the mind of the patient. A DNR order does not mean remove a ventilator. DNR just means no cardiopulmonary resuscitation efforts in the event of the patient's death.

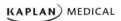

If the advance directive is not clear, particularly concerning basic nutrition, then you should continue therapy until it becomes clear. If you think that what is best for the patient is to remove the ventilator and he dies, what happens when you find out that the Alzheimer's disease is mild memory impairment and "no heroic measures" in the patient's mind meant no chemotherapy or surgery? Continue therapy until the situation is clear. In absence of a specific directive to stop, you should continue.

Definition of Health-Care Proxy

100. (c) To communicate and carry out the wishes of the patient

The health-care proxy is the agent of the patient to carry out the patient's wishes for their medical treatment in the event that she loses the capacity to make decisions for herself. The proxy is not an agent of the physician. The proxy should be the primary person to be the substitute for the judgment of the patient. In other words, what would the patient want if she were able to speak? The reason it is called a health-care proxy is to distinguish it from a financial executor. The power of the health-care proxy has no impact on the finances of the patient. They do not pay the bills for the patient.

The most important issue is that the primary role of the health-care agent or proxy is not there to state what the proxy thinks is best for the patient, but what the patient wanted. The proxy is like a mail carrier. If the patient's wishes are like a letter to the physician, the proxy is there to deliver it.

Pregnant Adult with Capacity

101. (a) Honor her wishes; no transfusion.

The pregnancy has no impact on the ability of a competent adult's right to refuse therapy. As long as the fetus is inside her body, the fetus does not have the independent rights of a person. The fetus is considered the same as her body. Personhood for the fetus is only a consideration after the delivery. The same answer would be true even if she were in her third trimester of pregnancy. The consent of the father is irrelevant. The father is not the one receiving the transfusion. Do not seek his opinion. The courts cannot order a competent person to receive a medical therapy she is refusing.

Oral Advance Directives Are Binding

102. (e) Remove the IV lines and stop blood draws as they wish.

There is no limitation on what can be withdrawn from a patient's care based on a clear advance directive. In this case the advance directive is oral. A written advance directive is preferable because it is easier to prove. This is especially important when there is disagreement amongst the family members. In this case, the wife and eight children are in uniform agreement on what the patient stated he wanted for himself. There is no ethical or legal distinction between withholding and withdrawing care.

An ethics committee is important when there is disagreement on what the patient's wishes were. Judicial intervention would be necessary if the physicians disagreed with the prognosis of the patient. In other words, if the family wanted everything stopped because they believed there would be no recovery but the physicians believed the impairment was temporary, then judicial intervention for a court order might be necessary.

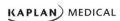

NOTES

NOTES

NOTES

NOTES

NOTES

NOTES

NOTES

NOTES

NOTES

NOTES

NOTES

NOTES

Boost your Step 3 score with Kaplan!

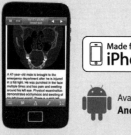
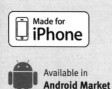

Made for iPhone

Available in **Android Market**

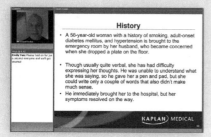

ALL NEW USMLE Step 3 Qbank

✓ Over a thousand exam-like questions written and approved by Dr. Conrad Fischer, Kaplan Medical's renowned instructor and one of the most experienced educators in medicine today

✓ Page references to this book, *Master the Boards USMLE® Step 3*: Cross-reference questions with book topics for deeper understanding

✓ NEW integrated mobile app: Turn downtime into a higher score—complete Qbank questions on your iPhone® or Android™ device

USMLE Step 3 Classroom Anywhere

Ideal for students in need of comprehensive review and a flexible study schedule.

✓ Over 90 hours of live lectures delivered by Dr. Conrad Fischer and other top Kaplan Medical faculty in an interactive, online classroom

✓ Real-time access to instructors and physician teaching assistants—have your questions answered on the spot

✓ Access to Kaplan's Step 3 online video library up to 30 days before and 60 days after lectures

✓ 3-volume Step 3 Lecture Notes, plus a pre-study diagnostic exam and 5 subject-based assessment tests

✓ Step 3 Qbank with free mobile app for the iPhone® or Android™ devices

Live Internal Medicine Board Review	✓ Over 54 hours of on-site, live instruction led by Dr. Conrad Fischer
	✓ Intense exposure to the challenges of patient management central to IM Board certification and fundamental to mastery on UMSLE Step 3
	✓ Dr. Fischer's comprehensive Internal Medicine Lecture Notes
	✓ Two months of access to IM Qbank (750 exam-style questions)
Live Online Internal Medicine Review	✓ 44 hours of live instruction led by Dr. Conrad Fischer in an interactive, online classroom—access from anywhere you have internet access
	✓ Real-time access to physician teaching assistants—have your questions answered on the spot
	✓ Access to lecture archives for 10 days from the end of the course
	✓ Dr. Fischer's comprehensive Internal Medicine Lecture Notes
	Learn more at: kaplanmedical.com/internalmedicine

To enroll or for more information, call 1-800-KAP-TEST or visit us at kaplanmedical.com/step3.

Coming in April 2013: Master the Wards

 Facebook.com/KaplanMedical   @kaplanmedical   Youtube.com/KaplanMedical09

1-800-KAP-TEST | kaplanmedical.com/step3

*USMLE is a joint program of The Federation of State Medical Boards of the United States, Inc. and the National Board of Medical Examiners. 10USML0211

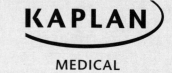

KAPLAN) MEDICAL